EUTHANASIA AND PALLIATIVE CARE
IN THE LOW COUNTRIES

ETHICAL PERSPECTIVES MONOGRAPH SERIES

3

Euthanasia and Palliative Care in the Low Countries

Editors

Paul Schotsmans
Tom Meulenbergs

PEETERS
LEUVEN – PARIS – DUDLEY, MA
2005

Library of Congress Cataloging-in-Publication Data

Euthanasia and palliative care in the Low Countries / editors, Paul Schotsmans,
Tom Meulenbergs.
    p. cm. -- (Ethical perspectives monograph series ; 3)
    Includes bibliographical references.
    ISBN 90-429-1556-0 (alk. paper)
    1. Euthanasia--Moral and ethical aspects--Benelux countries. 2. Euthanasia--Law
and legislation--Benelux countries. 3. Assisted suicide--Moral and ethical aspects--
Benelux Countries. 4. Assisted suicide--Law and legislation--Benelux countries.
5. Palliative treatment--Benelux countries. I. Schotsmans, Paul. II. Meulenbergs, Tom.
III. Series.

R726.E7865 2005
179.7'0942--dc22

                                                                                2004059520

ISBN 90-429-1556-0
D. 2005/0602/4

© 2005, Peeters – Bondgenotenlaan 153 – B-3000 Leuven – Belgium

TABLE OF CONTENTS

INTRODUCTION
EUTHANASIA AND PALLIATIVE CARE IN THE LOW COUNTRIES

Tom Meulenbergs & Paul Schotsmans

Belgium and the Netherlands — the Low Countries — are the first countries in the world that have legalized euthanasia. Since September 2002, Belgian physicians can perform euthanasia without at the same time performing a criminal act and in the Netherlands, the 'Termination of Life on Request and Assisted Suicide (Review Procedures) Act' came into force on the first of April 2002. For some, the Low Countries have become a shining example, for others the Belgian and Dutch legislations of end-of-life decision-making are the lamentable materializations of a culture of death. How diverse these reactions may be, their extreme character indicates that the Low Countries' end-of-life legislation is the subject of intense debate. This edited collection of papers is therefore conceived as an introduction to the legal and ethical debate surrounding the Belgian and Dutch Euthanasia Acts.

To engage in an informed debate, Maurice Adams and Herman Nys proceed with a detailed description and careful comparison of the both pieces of legislation. Despite the fact that within a period of less than one year Belgium and the Netherlands legalized euthanasia, the comparative study of Adams and Nys indicates that the Belgian and Dutch Act differ considerably. One of the most noticeable differences is their difference in length. Adams and Nys argue that this difference is due to the long established and legally accepted practice concerning euthanasia in the Netherlands whereas in Belgium no case law on the matter existed which obliged the Belgian legislator to write a far more detailed Euthanasia Act in order to guarantee maximum legal certainty for both physician and patient. With regard to the Euthanasia Act's material scope of application they indicate another significant difference: the Dutch Act explicitly includes physician assisted suicide while it remains unclear whether the Belgian Act is also applicable in these cases.

The situation in Belgium and the Netherlands diverges not only with regard to the material scope of the law. There also seems to be an important difference in the degree to which organized palliative care was involved in the debate that led to the establishment of the Euthanasia Act. That can be concluded from the contribution of Bert Broeckaert and Rien Janssens. They present an extensive description of how palliative care organizations have participated in the Dutch and Belgian euthanasia debate. While in Belgium organized palliative care was able to become one of the main actors in the debate, their Dutch counterparts felt prey to the fact that the Dutch debate had already been settled when they entered the public arena.

Law-making with respect to euthanasia is one thing. Bringing the law into practice is somewhat different. The question arises to what extent the new legal situation will bear upon the medical practice. Particularly, the responses of physicians are difficult to assess in advance. Physicians face the dilemma to report or not to report. They can take up their responsibility and report their practices of euthanasia, thereby exposing themselves to critical examination and possibly criminal prosecution. On the other hand, the physician can opt for safety and decide not to report his involvement in one of his patients' euthanasia. In the latter case, the introduction of new legislation would have missed the mark. To this day, the only available data with regard to physicians' reactions to an established legal framework wherein euthanasia is legalized come from the Netherlands. Since the vote on the law in 2000 and the establishment of 'regional review committees for termination of life on request and assisted suicide' in 2001, the reporting of euthanasia has declined. In their contribution Marta van Dijk, Guy Widdershoven and Agnes Meershoek examine this reporting procedure from a physician's perspective.

In the Netherlands the debate on end-of-life legislation took more than twenty years and the subsequent law on euthanasia reflected an existing medical practice. In his contribution, Guy Widdershoven argues that the Dutch debate — and by now Dutch practice — cannot be reduced to the "principlist canon of autonomy and beneficence". He claims, instead, that the values of responsibility, deliberation and care are central to Dutch euthanasia practice. In Belgium, on the contrary, Parliament eventually came to vote on a Euthanasia Bill after only half a decade of debate.

Besides factual presentations, this volume also includes some essays where end-of-life decision-making is discussed in more abstract terms. Daniel Sulmasy offers an exhaustive analysis of the notion of human dignity that constantly arises in debates on euthanasia and end-of-life decision-making. We examine whether the quality-of-life and sanctity-of-life ethics can be reconciled and Roger Burggraeve develops a foundational view on responsible care for dying people that should function as an alternative for the procedural way in which terminal care often is approached. The basis of his approach is the notion of 'responsibility-through-and-for-the-other' that comes from the moral philosophy of Emmanuel Levinas.

For Christian churches and Catholic healthcare institutions, the recent legalization of euthanasia and physician assisted suicide has proven to be challenging. Jan Jans describes the way in which the main Christian churches in Belgium and the Netherlands engaged in the debate and reacted to the eventual legalization. Chris Gastmans discusses the clinical practice guideline that was developed by Caritas Catholica Flanders, a Flemish Christian inspired umbrella organization for cooperation and consultation in health care and public welfare. This clinical practice guideline starts from the assumption that the fields of medicine, ethics and law are intertwined and that, apart from the legal provisions of the Euthanasia Act, a wider ethical framework is desirable in order to guarantee that people can die a humane death. This collection of essays concludes with a commentary of Herman De Dijn in which he holds a plea for authentic pluralism, which implies that a society should safeguard the possibility to organize health care from a specific philosophical or religious tradition.

We hope that the data, clarification and critical approaches on 'Euthanasia and Palliative Care in the Low Countries' presented in this volume shed more light on the development of a practice, which some still consider as non-medical behaviour and that these contributions may function as a catalyst for further debate on end-of-life decision-making.

Leuven, August 2004.

EUTHANASIA IN THE LOW COUNTRIES COMPARATIVE REFLECTIONS ON THE BELGIAN AND DUTCH EUTHANASIA ACT

Maurice Adams & Herman Nys

Introduction

On 28 May 2002, the *Act Concerning Euthanasia* (Euthanasia Act)[1] was passed by the Belgian House of Representatives, the lower house of parliament. A year before, the Belgian Senate had also approved the Act. On 23 September 2002, the Act came into force. This brought to an end a relatively brief legislative process that had begun in the summer of 1999.[2] That the Euthanasia Act emerged so quickly is all the more noteworthy given that the legislative process was in no way legally pre-structured: there existed no relevant case law and until very recently the public prosecutor's office had never initiated proceedings against anyone. Because of this, it was not known, for example, whether the concept of the so-called 'state of necessity',[3] as had

---

[1] For an English translation of the Belgian Euthanasia Act, see *Appendix I* in this volume, pp. 245-254.

[2] On this M. ADAMS, 'Euthanasia: the Process of Legal Change in Belgium. Reflections on the Parliamentary Debate' in A. KLIJN, M. OTLOWSKI & M. TRAPPENBURG (eds.), *Regulating Physician-Negotiated Death*, The Hague, Elsevier, 2001, pp. 29-47.

[3] The concept of the state of necessity can be invoked by a person who finds himself in a situation of a conflict of duties. If the person chooses to prefer the value that from an objective point of view is more important, even if this means doing something that in itself is forbidden, his conduct is legally justifiable. The two conflicts in case of euthanasia are of course the protection of life on the one hand, and the obligation to relieve the suffering of the patient on the other hand.

The concept seems to exist in almost all countries. In the United Kingdom, Glanville Williams has in 1957 already pointed to something similar as being a 'solution' for euthanasia, although he didn't believe it would be accepted by English judges in this context. G. WILLIAMS, *The Sanctity of Life and the Criminal Law*, New York, Knopf, 1957, p. 322.

been accepted by the Dutch Supreme Court ('Hoge Raad') in the context of euthanasia, would also be applicable in Belgium. This led to a situation where physicians were extremely uncertain of their legal situation, and from this point of view there was need for legislation. However, since 2000, the public prosecutor did begin to investigate cases of possible euthanasia. In January 2000, following reports by nursing personnel, two physicians (a cardiologist and an anaesthetist) in the city of Liège were arrested on suspicion of administering lethal barbiturates, at his own request and in consultation with his family, to a man suffering from a long-term chronic lung condition. On 6 February 2003 the Criminal Court of Liège decided not to prosecute both physicians, because under the Euthanasia Act — which then had come into force — their behaviour could not be considered an offence.

All this is in sharp contrast to the situation in the Netherlands where the recent Termination of Life on Request and Assisted Suicide (Review Procedures) Act,[4] which came into force on 1 April 2002, is generally considered to be a summary *codification* of accepted case law concerning euthanasia and assisted suicide. The Dutch case law has evolved over some 25 years along with the profession (physicians), patients' organizations, the public prosecutors' office, advisory bodies, etc.[5] Whereas the law in Belgium is intended primarily to *modify* physicians' behaviour by way of a political process,[6] in the Netherlands this was clearly not the case. One of the consequences of this difference is that in the Netherlands one can appeal to a qualitatively and quantitatively significant amount of case law and legal doctrine when interpreting the legislation. In Belgium, this is not

---

[4] For an English translation of the Dutch Euthanasia Act, see *Appendix II* in this volume, pp. 255-264.

[5] See on this H. WEYERS, 'Euthanasia: the Process of Legal Change in The Netherlands. The Making of Requirements of Careful Practice' in A. KLIJN, M. OTLOWSKI & M. TRAPPENBURG (eds.), *Regulating Physician-Negotiated Death*, pp. 1-27; J. GRIFFITHS, A. BOOD & H. WEYERS, *Euthanasia and Law in the Netherlands*, Amsterdam, Amsterdam University Press, 1998.

[6] It is not certain whether the Belgian legislature will succeed in this, since the Act seems to lack broad-based support among physicians themselves. A survey ordered by the Belgian *Journal du Médecin/Artsenkrant* (*i.e.* a bi-weekly journal for physicians), showed that only 42 percent of the physicians polled were willing to perform euthanasia conditionally, and only 15 percent would perform euthanasia on patients who would not die within a foreseeable period of time. *Market Analysis & Synthesis* (2001), pp. 6-9.

possible. As a result, a great deal of caution must be exercised when interpreting the Belgian Euthanasia Act, which is even more the case since the parliamentary debates sometimes lacked clarity.

It is precisely the lack of case law in Belgium that is one of the reasons why the Belgian Act, unlike the Dutch Act, contains so many detailed provisions. This is not merely an empirical observation. Although non-compliance with the conditions explicitly stipulated in both Acts can lead to criminal proceedings, in the Netherlands many detailed conditions of 'the law' of euthanasia and assisted suicide are not defined in the recent Act, but are rather concretized in case law or by norms generally accepted by the medical profession. In principle, such conditions have only disciplinary consequences.[7]

In this chapter we attempt two things: first, to compare the respective Belgian and Dutch Acts concerning euthanasia (with a focus on the Belgian Act) and, secondly, to situate the differences between them in a broader (mainly political) context. The latter is of course always important in any study of law. But particularly in the case of the Belgian Euthanasia Act, there would seem to be good reasons to invoke part of its political context, explicating some of the (sometimes surprising) choices that were made by the legislator.

1. The Material Scope of Application

1.1. *Euthanasia*

Section 2 of the Belgian Act defines euthanasia as the "intentional life-terminating action by someone other than the person concerned, at the request of the latter". The Belgian Advisory Committee on Bioethics had previously proposed this definition in its recommendation of 12 May 1997, regarding "The desirability of a legal regulation of euthanasia".[8] This Committee was established in 1993

---

[7] Of course, this does not preclude that case law dealing with the conditions of application explicitly concerned with the meaning of Dutch Act can also have consequences in criminal proceedings.

[8] The text of this recommendation can be consulted in Dutch and French at *http://www.health.fgov.be/bioeth/*. For an English translation of this recommendation, see H. Nys, 'Advice of the Federal Advisory Committee on Bioethics concerning legalization of euthanasia' in *European Journal of Health Law* 4(1997), pp. 389-393. On the recommendation itself, see J. Jans, 'Euthanasiegesetzgebung in Belgien. Eine Übersicht über die politisch-ethische Debatte 1997-1999' in A. Bondolfi & S. Grotenfeld

following years of political wrangling, and only officially installed in 1996. Its mandate is to provide advice and information to society and governmental authorities on problems which arise "as a result of research and its application in the fields of biology, medicine and health care ... The ethical, social and legal aspects of these problems are investigated, particularly as regards human rights" (according to section 1 of the committee's founding statutes). The Committee comprises 35 members — physicians, lawyers, ethicists, psychologists and sociologists — who are appointed with a view to linguistic and ideological parity, as is the custom in Belgium. One of the most important features of the Committee's recommendation is that it established for the first time in Belgium a clear, strict and authoritative definition of euthanasia, thus fulfilling a condition *sine qua non* for any meaningful social-political or legal debate about regulating euthanasia. The definition had its origin in a 1985 Dutch state commission on euthanasia, and had already been suggested in 1977 by a leading Dutch health care lawyer, Henk Leenen. Interestingly, the Dutch Act itself contains no definition of euthanasia, nor is the term mentioned in the Act. The Dutch Euthanasia Act only refers to termination of life by request, without explicitly defining this concept. However, based simply on the use of the phrase 'termination of life *by request*' and the Dutch Act's application conditions, it is clear that the scope of application of the two Acts is identical, at least in this respect. Moreover, section 293 §1 of the Dutch Criminal Code contains a crime that strongly resembles the Belgian definition of euthanasia: "A person who terminates the life of another person at that other person's express and earnest request is liable to a term of imprisonment of not more than twelve years or a fine of the fifth category."

1.2. *Assisted suicide*

The Belgian Euthanasia Act, in contrast to its Dutch counterpart, does not apply to assisted suicide. This is surprising, since it is generally accepted that the differences between euthanasia on the one hand and assisted suicide on the other, are ethically irrelevant, or at least minimal. So it would be logical for both types of action to be tied to the same legal standard. Why regulate the 'greater' but not the

(eds.), *Ethik und Gesetzgebung. Probleme — Lösungsversuche — Konzepte*, Stuttgart, Verlag W. Kolhammer, 2000, pp. 175-187.

'lesser'? Nevertheless it *seems* that the Belgian legislature made this choice deliberately, in spite of the fact that advice by the Belgian Council of State in respect to the Bill, strongly criticized this choice.

One reason for this exclusion might be that, unlike section 294 of the Dutch Criminal Code, Belgian criminal law does not make suicide a punishable offence. One could then argue that assisting suicide can also not be considered a crime, which would obviate the need for regulation. This line of argument is, however, not entirely convincing. There are some who believe that assisted suicide might indeed be a punishable offence in an indirect way. They invoke section 422 of the Belgian Criminal Code concerning negligence for failing to assist a person in grave danger. The assumption is that a person wishing to commit suicide must be prevented from doing so, since he, or she, is in grave danger. In the absence of any Belgian case law, however, there is no clear way of knowing whether this line of reasoning is sound.

In addition, from the point of view of patient autonomy, assisted suicide is actually preferable to euthanasia. The former offers more safeguards from abuse, since suicide is carried out by the patient him/herself. In any case, respect for patient autonomy is a problem in Flanders, since a recent study on medical decisions regarding the end of life, shows that there is a relatively high rate of direct termination of life without an explicit request by the patient. This sort of action occurred almost three times more frequently than euthanasia. Euthanasia is only the tip of the iceberg, constituting 1,1 percent of the total number of deaths studied, whereas related actions such as assisted suicide and direct termination of life without the patient's request occurred in 0,1 percent and 3,2 percent, respectively, of deaths studied.[9] It seems there is a problem here with freedom of choice and patient autonomy.

In our opinion the most likely explanation for the exclusion of assisted suicide is concerned with the ideological and political context within which the legislative process in Belgium was played out. From the very beginning of the parliamentary process, a hostile atmosphere prevailed between the government and opposition parties. Proponents and opponents of the bill did not hesitate from portraying each other as extremists (conservative or liberal) in the interests of political image formation. In this context, from the very

---

[9] L. DELIENS *et al.*, 'End-of-life Decisions in Medical Practice in Flanders, Belgium' in *The Lancet* 356(2000), pp. 1806-1811.

beginning of the debate, the term 'assisted suicide' for a great many members of Parliament came to mean literally simply killing someone at their request with no additional conditions. It should be obvious that in particular the proponents of the Bill did not want to be accused of supporting something so 'frivolous'. The fact that the distinction between the two Acts lies only in the way the physician goes about his work, was at a certain moment no longer relevant for many of those involved.[10] One of the politicians who intervened on this issue on several occasions in the Belgian Senate noticed this misunderstanding and submitted amendments, but they were all rejected. The time for making choices had passed, and the Bill's approval, according to politicians from the governing coalition, would no longer be delayed.

Yet it is quite possible that in making this distinction between euthanasia and assisted suicide, the Belgian Act is discriminatory in an unconstitutional way. The Belgian constitutional court (the 'Arbitragehof') could accordingly judge this discrimination to be in contravention of the sections 10 and 11 of the Belgian constitution, incorporating, respectively, the principles of non-discrimination and equality. The regular courts might also be able to provide a solution. If a judge is of the opinion that only the letter of the law can be employed in making an interpretation, then a physician who assists a suicide on the same conditions as are applicable to euthanasia is out of luck: he or she will face criminal charges. However, if the judge applies a more constructive or teleological interpretation of the Belgian Act, seeking inspiration in the Act's preparatory documents, then he or she will quickly discover that there has been a mistake and that the actual intention was not so much to exclude assisted suicide, but rather to exclude totally free euthanasia. In any case, as far as we are concerned, the choice made by the Belgian legislature is not convincing.[11]

1.3. *Other end-of-life decisions*

Neither the Dutch nor the Belgian Act deals with any other end-of-life decision than euthanasia. This has attracted some criticism: since

---

[10] Particularly the Parliamentary Proceedings of the committee discussions in the Belgian Senate is filled with examples of such confusions of language.

[11] Unless the context indicates otherwise, in what follows, we also include assisted suicide when speaking of euthanasia, as far as the Netherlands is concerned.

euthanasia can be camouflaged as pain control, any official supervision of euthanasia is impossible as long as not all end-of-life decisions and actions are regulated.[12] The question is whether such broad supervision is viable in practice, since it would possibly lead to an unmanageable bureaucracy that defeats its purpose. The best way of remedying this would seem to be by guaranteeing patient autonomy through the enactment of legislation on patients' rights.[13]

2. The Personal Scope of Application

2.1. *The physician*

According to sections 3 §1 and 4 §2 of the Belgian Act, the physician who performs euthanasia commits no offence when he or she complies with the norms and procedures stipulated in the Act. In the Netherlands, the situation is somewhat different: section 293 §1 of the Dutch Criminal Code (as amended by section 20 of the Dutch Euthanasia Act), states that ending someone's life at their request remains a criminal offence, but that the physician who respects the criteria laid down in section 2 of the Dutch Euthanasia Act and who reports to the municipal coroner in accordance with section 7, second §of the so-called Cremation and Burials Act, may legitimately rely on section 293 §2 of the Dutch Criminal Code. This means that the crime continues to exist, but the physician is not punishable. The result, technically speaking, is that there is in the Netherlands no decriminalization of euthanasia. As far as the burden of proof is concerned it makes no difference which option, the Belgian or Dutch, is taken: both in the Netherlands and in Belgium, the public prosecutor bears the burden of proving that, in cases such as this, a criminal offence is committed.

In both Belgium and the Netherlands, only a *physician* can legitimately perform euthanasia. In Belgium, no further requirements are imposed on the physician's competence: the physician performing euthanasia does not have to be the attending physician, nor is any

---

[12] See on this extensively, GRIFFITHS, J., A. BOOD & H. WEYERS, *Euthanasia and Law in the Netherlands*, pp. 259-298.

[13] Such an Act recently came into force in Belgium, *i.e.* the Act of 22 August 2002 concerning patients' rights.

special expertise required, for instance, in palliative care. The latter is not required in the Netherlands either. However, in the Netherlands it is generally accepted that the physician who performs euthanasia should *in principle* be the attending physician.[14] In fact, in 70 percent of cases it is the patient's general practitioner.[15] In this context, Griffiths makes reference to the so-called 'travelling euthanasia doctors' — responsible for a slight fuss in 1994 — who became involved with euthanasia via the 'Dutch Society of Voluntary Euthanasia', in cases where the patient's own doctor refused to perform it.[16] Given the fact that, on the one hand, a significant number of Belgian physicians appear not to support the Euthanasia Act[17] and, on the other hand, the capacity of the attending physician is not explicitly required, one can expect that Belgian euthanasia practice is more 'vulnerable' to such 'travelling euthanasia doctors'. Perhaps the 'attending physician' requirement can be derived implicitly from section 3 of the Belgian Act, where it is stipulated that the physician must have a number of conversations with the patient, spread over a reasonable period of time, in order to be certain of the durability of the euthanasia request. In addition, a balanced assessment of the legal requirements demands some familiarity with the patient and his or her symptoms. Against this, however, one can read in the parliamentary documents that a patient should be able to completely exclude his attending physician from the decision-making process. The situation is not, therefore, altogether clear.

It is noteworthy that the Belgian Act, unlike the Dutch Act, does not specify which offence is committed by the physician when he or she fails to comply with the norms and procedures established by the Act. This is all the more striking since the Belgian Act — once again unlike section 293 of the Dutch Criminal Code — has never recognized euthanasia as a separate offence.

---

[14] Griffiths points out that no specific source *in law* can be found for this generally accepted principle. J. GRIFFITHS, A. BOOD & H. WEYERS, *Euthanasia and Law in the Netherlands*, p. 103, note 41. It is, however, a generally accepted guideline of good practice, as found in many reports and documents drafted by advisory bodies and physicians' organizations.

[15] H.J.J. LEENEN, 'The development of euthanasia in the Netherlands' in *European Journal of Health Law* 8(2001), p.128.

[16] GRIFFITHS, J., A. BOOD & H. WEYERS, *EUTHANASIA AND LAW IN THE NETHERLANDS*, p. 103, note 41. With the necessary reservations, this practice is nevertheless considered acceptable by some Dutch district courts.

[17] See note 9 above.

The question thus arises: what offence does the physician in Belgium actually commit when not legitimately committing euthanasia? Is it manslaughter,[18] murder[19] or poisoning?[20] This uncertainty is only exasperated by the fact that, until recently, no prosecutions for euthanasia had taken place and there exists no case law on the matter. The reason for this state of affairs probably has to do with the fact that the (conditional) decriminalization of euthanasia in Belgium was not implemented through the Criminal Code but by means of a separate act, thereby leaving the Criminal Code unaltered. This choice, however, was made only after the legislative process had been underway for some time in Parliament. Changing the situation would have meant a considerable delay, which was politically not acceptable to the majority parties in Parliament. In any case, with the construction ultimately chosen — namely no alteration of the Criminal Code but the introduction of a separate act on the matter — it is emphasized by the legislature that the protection of life is and remains a matter of principle, and that killing by request is not a 'normal' affair. But whatever the reason may have been for this choice, unfortunately the question of what provision of the Criminal Code is violated when the conditions of performing euthanasia are not met was left open. In our opinion, this omission represents an infringement of the principle of legality in criminal law.

Continuing along these lines, the Belgian Euthanasia Act also makes no distinction between criminalization in cases of serious or less serious infringements of the Act. Thus, even bearing in mind the possibility of invoking mitigating circumstances, ignoring a merely formal requirement, such as for example not completing the necessary documents in the proper way, might lead to a sanction being imposed which can scarcely be said to stand in a reasonable proportion to the facts. In this sense, proportionality is lost.

An interesting issue concerns the question regarding the conclusion to be drawn from the fact that only a physician may perform euthanasia. Among healthcare lawyers in the Netherlands, the majority seem to be of the opinion that euthanasia is nevertheless not a 'standard medical act', but a socially regulated act in which physicians happen to be involved. Indeed, if euthanasia were a standard

[18] Belgian Criminal Code, section 292.
[19] *Ibid.*, section 394.
[20] *Ibid.*

medical act, then refusing to answer a patient's request when the legal requirements are met, would be in conflict with the physician's professional duty.[21] There is more discussion surrounding this in Belgium. Some believe that it is indeed a standard medical act, and the fact that a *physician* must perform euthanasia is cited as proof of this. This argument is unpersuasive: the fact that euthanasia must be performed by a physician does indeed mean that we are dealing with an act carried out by a medical professional, but that does not yet make it a *standard* medical act. Moreover, if it were indeed a standard medical act, then the requirement that a physician must perform euthanasia would be superfluous, since in Belgium this requirement would follow anyway from legislation regulating the activities of healthcare professionals. In any event, based on section 14 of the Belgian Euthanasia Act, the physician is not required to consent to a patient's request for euthanasia, which means that there does not exist something like a (subjective) right to euthanasia. Once again, the key to understanding this issue lies in the political context, and ultimately involves the question of whether specifically Catholic hospitals may prohibit physicians working within their walls from performing euthanasia. The answer to this is not merely academic, since about 80 percent of the hospitals in Flanders are associated with Catholic organizations.[22]

Contrary to what is the case in the Netherlands, in Belgium there is no legal requirement for the physician to use 'due medical care' when performing euthanasia.[23] Though there was debate on this point in Parliament, the governing parties considered the requirement to be superfluous since a physician is always required to exercise due medical care. Whether this was an accurate assessment is nevertheless open to question. In any case, it is apparent from Dutch

---

[21] In the Netherlands, this debate took place primarily in the context of the question whether the so-called 'medical exception' should be applicable in the case of euthanasia. The concept of the 'medical exception' means that although the Criminal Code does not contain exceptions for medical behaviour, it is nevertheless not criminal as long as it is being done within the margins of normal medical acts. The Dutch Supreme Court rejected the request for the medical expection to be applicable to euthanasia. See its judgement of 21 October 1986, *Nederlandse Jurisprudentie* 1987, no. 607.

[22] For the position statement of Caritas Catholica, the umbrella organization of Catholic healthcare institutions in the Dutch-speaking part of Belgium, on euthanasia, see the contribution of Chris Gastmans in this volume, pp. 205-225.

[23] Dutch Euthanasia Act, section 2 §1(e).

disciplinary case law that a duty of due medical care in cases of euthanasia imposes a number of specific requirements. For instance, the Medical Disciplinary College of Amsterdam decided on 11 April 1994 that a physician must remain with the patient until such a time as death has been established, or else that he must be available at very short notice in order to intervene if needed. In addition, the physician must administer the necessary lethal medication in the correct dosage, which is perhaps one of the most important aspects of the due care requirement for euthanasia.

Finally, the physician in Belgium does not have to consent to a euthanasia request; he may refuse to perform euthanasia on grounds of conscience or for medical reasons.[24] In such a case, however, he must inform the patient or any person representing the patient (see below), within a reasonable time, and explain the reasons for refusal. If the physician's refusal is based on medical grounds, then it must be noted in the patient's medical record. Moreover, at the request of the patient or representative, the physician who refuses to fulfil a request for euthanasia must hand over the patient's medical record to the physician appointed by the patient or the representative. Indeed, the physician may also make his willingness to consent to a request for euthanasia subject to additional conditions, as is provided by section 3 §2 and 4 §2. The physician in the Netherlands may also refuse to fulfil a request for euthanasia. The Dutch parliamentary proceedings — though not the Dutch Act itself — establish that in such a case a duty exists to refer the patient to another physician.

2.2. *The patient*

The Belgian Act requires that to make a legitimate request for euthanasia an individual must have attained the age of majority (18 or older). In general, minors are excluded from the Belgian Euthanasia Act, which results from the fact that the subject was so controversial that including it would have threatened overall approval of the Act. From this perspective, the Dutch Act is completely different, as can be seen from section 2, §3 and 4 of the Act. If a minor aged between 16 and 18 is deemed to have a reasonable understanding of his own interests in the matter, then he can submit a legitimate request for euthanasia, at least if the parent(s) or the legal

---

[24] Belgian Euthanasia Act, section 14.

guardian who exercises authority over the minor is included in the decision process. Moreover, if a minor patient aged between 12 and 16 is deemed to have a reasonable understanding of his own interests in the matter, then the physician may consent to the minor patient's request if the parent(s) or guardian who exercises authority over the minor is able to reconcile themselves with the request.

3. The Patient's Request

An important aspect of both Acts has to do with the patient's request. The Belgian Act draws a distinction between a request in the strict sense (section 3) and a request by means of an advance directive (section 4). The Dutch Act also makes this distinction, but as far as the latter is concerned refers to a 'written declaration'. To facilitate comparison, we will refer to the former type of request as the 'current request' and to the latter as the 'advance directive'.

3.1. *The current request*

The Belgian Act regulates in detail the formal and material requirements for a current request. Pursuant to section 3 §1, such a request must be 'voluntary', 'considered' and 'repeated'; moreover, it must not be the result of any external pressure. Section 3 §1, 2 further stipulates that the physician must verify that the request is 'durable', ascertaining this by means of several discussions. Note that the Act does not say the request must be *well informed*, though this is perhaps entailed by the requirement that it be 'considered': a request can only be considered when the patient has arrived at the request after weighing up all the elements, including all medical and other information. In principle, the request must also be written by the patient himself, which means drafted, dated and signed by the patient (section 3 §4), and retained in the patient's medical record (section 3 §5). If the patient is incapable of writing down the request, as a result of a disability for example, then it is to be written down by an adult person who has been chosen by the patient and who has no material interest in the patient's death, such as a relative of the patient. This person must record the fact that the patient is not able to formulate the request in writing, and refers to the reasons why. In this case, the drafting of the request must take place in the presence of the physician, and the person must record the name of the physician in the document (these two people do not need to sign the document themselves). The document must be appended to the medical record. The patient may revoke the request at any time, which results in the document being removed from the medical record and returned to the patient (section 3 §4, final sentence).

The Dutch Act, by contrast, speaks only of a 'voluntary and well-considered' request (section 2(1)(a)), with no further formal requirements. In section 293 of the Dutch Criminal Code it is also stated that the request should be 'explicit and serious'. Compared to the Belgian Act, these are rather concise formulations. However, if we examine the due care criteria as they have been established primarily in some authoritative reports on euthanasia as written by advisory bodies and health care organizations, then Dutch euthanasia practice turns out to accept more onerous requirements than the Act would suggest. For instance, the request must in principle be expressed by the requesting party himself; it must be independent, in other words not resulting from any external pressure; it must be well-considered, which means well-informed, following consultations and based on a durable wish for the end of life (which can be demonstrated by the request having been repeated several times over a certain period of time). This latter criterion was expressly omitted as a criterion in the Dutch Act because it was thought that it might cause problems in situations of acute emergency. Finally, the request should preferably be drafted in writing or registered in some other way.

3.2. *The advance directive*

Section 4 §1 of the Belgian Act regulates in detail the formal requirements imposed on an advance directive in cases where a patient is no longer able to express his will. Interestingly, the material requirements imposed when it is a *current request* no longer apply here.

The advance directive may be drafted at any time. It must be set down in writing in the presence of two adult witnesses, at least one of whom has no material interest in the patient's death, and it must be dated and signed by the patient making the request, by the witnesses and by the patient's representative, if any. In the advance directive, one or more representatives may be appointed, in order of preference, who will inform the attending physician of the patient's wishes. In the event of refusal, hindrance, incapacity or death, each representative will be replaced by the person indicated in the advance directive. The patient's attending physician, the physician consulted (see below) and the members of the nursing team are prohibited from acting as persons taken in confidence. The advance directive may be modified or revoked at any time. Delegated legislation, which at the time of writing this chapter still has to be issued, determines the way in which the advance directive is best to be drafted, registered, reconfirmed or revoked and, through the office of the Central State Registry, how it is to be communicated to the physicians involved. There is, however no requirement to utilize the form in the way that will be provided for in that legislation. As a consequence, other forms of advance directive may also be legally valid.

If the patient who wishes to draft an advance directive is permanently physically incapable of doing so, he may appoint an adult who has no material interest in his death to write down his request, in the presence of two adult witnesses, at least one of whom has no material interest in the patient's death. The advance directive must note that the patient in question is incapable of signing and refers to the reasons why. The advance directive must be dated and signed by the person who writes it down, by the witnesses and by the representatives, if any. A medical certificate is appended to the advance directive as proof that the patient is permanently physically incapable of writing and signing the advance directive.

The Belgian legislature's objective of limiting the validity of the advance directive to five years following its drafting or confirmation cannot be attained with the Euthanasia Act in its current form, since the third last paragraph of section 4 §1 states: an advance directive is only valid 'if it has been drafted or confirmed less than 5 years before the moment at which the person in question can no longer express his wishes'. Consider a case where someone drafted such an advance directive on 1 January 1995. On 1 January 2003 the advance directive is then presented to a physician. How can this physician possibly know how long the person in question has been unable to express his wishes? It might be since 1996, but it might also be since 2002. In the former case, the advance directive would be valid since only one year had elapsed between drafting the advance directive and the moment of incapacity; in the latter case, the advance directive would be invalid. This problem could easily have been avoided by correctly formulating the Euthanasia Bill. In determining the advance directive's validity, what is crucial is not the moment at which patients can no longer express their wishes, but rather the moment at which the advance directive's execution is requested. If more than five years has elapsed between drafting or confirming the advance directive and the moment at which its execution is requested, it should no longer be considered valid. That would have been an objective, easily verifiable moment. One of the authors (H. Nys) drew attention to this problem during hearings on the Bill at the Belgian House of Representatives on 27 February 2002. The parliamentary representatives were aware of the problem but did not want to modify the text of the Bill, since this would have had constitutional consequences: had there been the slightest alteration to the text, then the Belgian Senate would have had to vote yet again on the modified version of the text. That would have taken too much time, and the government parties did not, for political reasons, want this to occur.

Section 2(2) of the Dutch Act stipulates that in cases of an advance directive, the due care criteria of section 2(1) apply, which means that the patient must have been capable of making a voluntary, well-considered request at the time the advance directive was drafted. As we have just seen with regard to the Belgian Act, no further legal requirements are imposed on an advance directive in Belgium. The law does not demand that there must be a voluntary, well-considered and repeated request, not resulting from external pressure, as is the case with a current request. This is a significant difference between the Belgian and Dutch legislation. The Dutch Act does not require the advance directive to have any specific formal qualities, apart from being drafted in writing. In any case, euthanasia as a consequence of an advance directive occurs very rarely in the Netherlands, and one reason for this is that before the Act was passed there were already doubts regarding the legal validity in general of such an instrument.[25] This might also explain why very few due care criteria on this issue are to be found in case law and authoritative reports. Even now that there is legislation allowing the use of an advanced directive, few expect that it will frequently be used.

---

[25] J. GRIFFITHS & A. KLIJN, 'Can doctors' hands be bound? Advance directives under current Dutch law', 1999. To be found at *http://ww.rechten.rug.nl/mbpsl/milaanpa.htm*.

4. The Patient's Situation

Another material requirement deals with the patient's state of health. Once again, we will distinguish between the two situations outlined in the preceding section, namely the situation where the patient submits a current request, and the situation where a request is made by means of an advance directive.

4.1. *The current request*

In section 3 §1 the Belgian Act stipulates that the physician must be certain that the patient who submits a current request is in a 'medically hopeless situation' characterized by 'persistent and unbearable physical or mental suffering which cannot be alleviated and which results from a serious and incurable condition caused by accident or illness'. This definition has provoked copious and confused debates in Parliament.

One can distinguish a more objective and a more subjective element in this. The more subjective element has to do with the *serious* and *incurable* nature of the condition caused by an accident or illness. We may assume that, in general, physicians possess the knowledge and expertise to decide about a condition's seriousness and incurability. The Belgian Act makes no distinction between conditions of a physical or a mental nature or origin. Terminal illness is therefore not required by the Belgian Act, nor is it a requirement that has ever been imposed by Dutch case law or the recent Dutch Act. Be that as it may, one of the arguments invoked during the Belgian legislative process for not imposing the requirement of terminal illness, is that it is impossible to define what exactly constitutes a terminal patient. This is, in our opinion, less than convincing: physicians are quite capable of determining what the average life expectancy will be of someone who is in a situation of a patient who submits a euthanasia request. That there can be no absolute certainty and that some patients will in fact live more or less longer than expected, does nothing to diminish this fact. Ultimately, then, this is a matter of reaching an agreement about what terminal means: is it three months, three weeks or three days?

Returning to the issue of a 'medically hopeless situation' characterized by 'persistent and unbearable physical or mental suffering which cannot be alleviated and which results from a serious and incurable condition caused by accident or illness'. Does, for instance, a person suffering from cancer who can be treated temporarily with intensive chemotherapy and thereby live one or two years longer fall under the Act? Maybe not; at least not on the face of it. However, the link with the fact that a medically hopeless situation can involve a purely subjective element — namely whether or not the illness can be alleviated — would seem, in Belgium at least, to render such an interpretation unimportant.

This is a consequence of two interpretative points. First, of the fact that it is the patient, and the patient alone, who determines whether he is suffering from persistent and unbearable physical or mental suffering. The physician's task is simply to be certain that *the patient* finds *himself* in such a situation. If the patient says that this is the case, then the physician can do little else but acknowledge this. There is nothing in the Act about the physician's interpretation or understanding of the concrete symptoms from which the patient is suffering nor about experience with pain and suffering of patients in comparable situations.

Secondly, the Belgian Act does not require a patient to undergo alternative treatment before the physician may consent to a euthanasia request. Indeed, section 3 §2, 1 stipulates only that the physician must *discuss* with the patient 'his request for euthanasia and any remaining therapeutic options, including that of palliative care …'. In our opinion, one *might* conclude from this combination of facts that the patient — for instance the cancer patient mentioned earlier — may refuse a treatment, whereby the patient ends up in a medically hopeless situation. As a consequence, the physician may legitimately agree to such a patient's euthanasia request. The sole objective requirement of the Act — of a serious and incurable condition caused by accident or illness — can as a result perhaps be subjectively fulfilled to a significant or even crucial degree.

Yet at the same time, it may of course also be the case that the general legal principles of subsidiarity and proportionality apply, despite the suggestion created by the text of the Act. Consenting to a request from a patient for whom there still exists a genuine treatment alternative could then constitute a non-subsidiary or disproportionate action on the part of the physician, since other treatment possibilities would still be open.

Unfortunately, the Belgian Act is not entirely clear on this aspect. In any event, if the 'liberal' interpretation of the Belgian Act is correct, then herein lies quite a significant difference with the Dutch Act — or rather with Dutch law. Again, the Dutch Act is much more concise in this regard. In section 2 §1(b), it stipulates that the physician must believe that the patient is suffering hopelessly and unbearably, and that, in addition, *together with the patient*, he must believe that there is no other reasonable solution to the situation in which the patient finds himself. So it is the physician, together with the patient, who must arrive at the belief that there is no other solution for the situation of the patient.

All this is accepted in Dutch case law,[26] where it is stated that the requirement of 'hopelessness' constitutes an objective element, or at least that its assessment lies with the physician(s) alone. The same is also true, for the requirement of 'unbearability'. As we just saw, this requirement is also not determined by the patient alone. So whereas the requirement of 'unbearability' in the Netherlands constitutes, at least in part, an objective element — it is a matter of medical irreversibility or hopelessness, depending on the professional opinion of a physician — in Belgium it seems that it is conceived as a wholly subjective element.

The Dutch 1994 *Chabot* case provides an illustration of the possible significance of this difference between the law in the Netherlands and Belgium. *Chabot* involved a woman who said she suffered 'hopelessly' and 'unbearably' as a result of psychiatric problems. Although in its judgement the Dutch Supreme Court in principle agreed that a psychiatric disorder can be a legitimate reason for assisted suicide, it also stated that:

> In assessing whether there is unbearable and hopeless suffering, such that providing assistance with suicide would be regarded as a justified choice in an emergency situation, it is important to bear in mind that *there can in principle be no question of hopelessness if a real alternative for alleviating that suffering has been freely refused by the person concerned* (emphasis added).[27]

Shortly after this ruling, the District Court of Haarlem followed the Supreme Court and pronounced judgement in the case of a man who, as a result of three strokes, was disabled on one side and who

---

[26] See in particular the 1984 *Schoonheim* decision by the Dutch Supreme Court, *Nederlandse Jurisprudentie* 1985, no. 106.

[27] Though the *Chabot* judgement pertains to assisted suicide with psychiatric patients, the ruling also applies to patients with purely physical complaints.

could not accept being a permanent invalid as a result. The judge ruled that one could not speak of hopeless suffering if a genuine alternative — psychiatric help in this case — for alleviating such suffering had been freely rejected by the patient. In other words, the physician was at fault for having too easily accepted the patient's refusal to explore other alternatives.

In both cases, the judge invoked the principle of subsidiarity (on which the concept of 'hopelessness' depends), and commentators seem to agree unanimously that assisted suicide cannot be justified in the case of a patient who refuses medically meaningful treatment.[28] Here we are confronted with a possible significant difference between the Belgian Act and Dutch law, a difference that results, provided that the liberal interpretation of the Belgian Act is correct, in the Belgian Act being the more liberal of the two, at least as far as this aspect is concerned.

It should also be noted that assisted suicide, as we saw earlier, does not fall within the Belgian Act. However, all Dutch case law regarding psychiatric patients concerns assisted suicide. This raises questions about comparability, since it leads to the paradoxical situation where euthanasia is applicable to psychiatric patients in Belgium, but assisted suicide is not. The chairman of the Commission of Justice in the Belgian House of Representatives — one of the commissions in which the euthanasia Bill was debated — concluded that euthanasia can never be an option in respect of a psychiatric patient, since mental suffering is irreconcilable with a voluntary and well-considered expression of one's wishes.[29] This opinion is not just in opposition to the Dutch Supreme Court in the *Chabot* case, but more particularly it seems to run counter to any meaningful interpretation of the words (and the intention) of the Belgian Euthanasia Act. In any event, it remains to be seen what the attitude of medical practitioners will be. In view of the Belgian physicians' conservative stance toward the

---

[28] J. GEVERS & J. LEGEMAATE, 'Physician assisted suicide in psychiatry: an analysis of case law and professional options' in D.C.THOMASMA *et al.* (eds.), *Asking to die. Inside the Dutch debate about euthanasia*, The Hague, Kluwer Academic Publishers, 1997, pp. 71-91.

[29] Incidentally, the Belgian House of Representatives' Committee on Public Health, which fulfilled an advisory role for the House Committee on Justice in this matter, unanimously recommended that mental suffering alone should never be able to legitimate euthanasia. None of the opinions of the Committee on Public Health was followed.

Euthanasia Act, one should not expect any major changes in practice. What remains, in any case, is an absence of legal certainty.

Finally, as we have seen, the text of the Belgian Act explicitly speaks of medical hopelessness as a consequence of 'a serious and incurable condition caused by *accident or illness*' (emphasis added). This means that the legislator apparently wanted to exclude so-called *Brongersma* situations from the Act's applicability. In its judgement of December 2002 the Dutch Supreme Court found, in the *Brongersma* case, that a request for assisted suicide or euthanasia should always be the result of a somatic illness. So although a person's request for assisted suicide or euthanasia can indeed be in a 'hopeless' and 'unbearable' situation, if he is not suffering from a psychiatric or physical *illness* (*i.e.* when there is no direct somatic cause for the wish to die) a physician cannot legitimately answer the request. Of course, the question then remains whether it is possible to clearly define the concept of 'illness' so as to utilise it in practice. This may not be possible, primarily due to the fact that it is usually not clear when a request to die is the result of someone merely being tired of living, or when such a request is also the result of a physical or mental condition. Most physicians seem to agree that in fact some reason can always be found on the basis of which a euthanasia request can be (partly) reduced to a somatic (physical or mental) cause. It could very well be, then, that the requirement contained in the Belgian Act is practically irrelevant.

4.2. *The advance directive*

The Belgian Act contains special requirements regarding the patient's state of health when he is no longer conscious where an advance directive exists. Section 4 §1 stipulates that such a patient must be suffering from a serious, incurable condition caused by accident or illness and, moreover, that the state of unconsciousness must be irreversible according to the current state of science. The requirement of unbearable suffering is no longer imposed, since the legislature assumed that such patients are no longer capable of suffering. Had this requirement been imposed, the fear was that euthanasia in cases of irreversibly unconscious patients would have been impossible. In spite of the Act leaving little room for interpretation as far as this aspect is concerned, most members of Parliament assumed that only patients in a so-called persistent vegetative state (PVS) would meet this criterion. Quite a lot of discussion nevertheless took place on this point in the Belgian Parliament. One of the members of Parliament who had submitted the legislative bill — the leader of the Dutch-speaking liberal party in the Senate — was of the opinion that, as far as she was concerned, the Act should apply mainly to comatose patients, which is broader than an 'irreversibly unconscious' patient. This gave rise to questions about the applicability of the Act to older people with dementia for instance: are they in irreversibly unconscious situations since they no longer possess any real powers of awareness? While most members of Parliament believed that this ought not to be the case, no definitive answer was ever given on this point. As a result, there exists a lack of clarity on this issue.

The Dutch Act, by contrast, states in section 2 §2 that an advance directive can be applied when the patient 'is no longer capable of expressing his wishes'. This requirement is clearly broader than the requirement of the Belgian Act (there is no mention of irreversible unconsciousness). The Act places no special requirements on the patient in cases of an advance directive, but only states, also in section 2 §2, that the 'requirements of due care referred to in the first paragraph apply *mutatis mutandis*'. In view of what has just been said, we might ask ourselves what this could mean with respect to the requirement of unbearable suffering? Can, for example, someone who is unconscious suffer unbearably? Because of this, commentators have raised doubts about the feasibility of this provision in practice.

5. Duties of the Physician with respect to the Patient's Request

5.1. *The current request*

The Belgian Act goes into great detail as far as this aspect is concerned. In section 3 §1 and §2, the Act stipulates that the physician who performs euthanasia does not commit a crime when he has made certain that the patient's situation is in accordance with the conditions laid down in the Act. In addition, section 3 §2 stipulates that the physician must in every case inform the patient beforehand about his state of health and his life expectancy, discuss with the patient his request for euthanasia, and discuss any remaining therapeutic options including those offered by palliative care, as well as their consequences. He must consult another physician regarding the serious and incurable nature of the condition, and inform him of the reason for such a consultation. The recommendation of the physician who is consulted is not binding, but such a consultation can of course be authoritative or even incriminating in the event of any later disputes. The physician consulted must be independent both of the patient and of the attending physician, and must be 'competent' to assess the condition in question.[30] He has to inspect the medical record, examine the patient and must make certain of the persistent and unbearable physical or mental suffering that cannot be alleviated. He also has to make a report on his findings. The attending physician must moreover inform the patient of the results of this consultation. In addition, if there is a nursing team in regular contact with the patient, then the patient's request must be discussed with that team or its members as well. Finally, should the patient so desire, the request must also be discussed with family or friends named by the patient. Of course, only the views of the patient himself are decisive; the opinions of the family and friends consulted are not definitive for the legitimacy of the act of euthanasia. Yet this does not preclude the physician from being influenced by the opinions of family and friends in deciding not to agree to a euthanasia request.

In the event that the attending physician believes the patient is not going to die within a foreseeable period of time, there are a number of additional requirements that he must fulfil: in the first place, section 3 §3 stipulates that he must consult a *second* physician, who is a psychiatrist or a specialist in the condition in question, and inform him of the reason for such a consultation. This second physician must also inspect the medical record, examine the patient and make certain of the persistent and unbearable physical or mental suffering which cannot be alleviated, as well as the voluntary, well-considered and repeated nature of the request. This physician must also report on his findings, and must be independent of the patient, of the attending physician and of the first physician consulted. In this case as well, the attending physician is obliged to inform the patient of the results of this consultation. Moreover, in the case of a non-terminal patient, at least one month must elapse between the patient's written request and the act of euthanasia.

A general requirement established by section 3 §5 is that all requests formulated by the patient, and all actions performed by

---

[30] In principle, every physician is *legally* competent, but the term is also used here in the sense of *professionally* competent. The French version of the Belgian Euthanasia Act uses the term 'compétent', which encompasses both meanings.

the attending physician and their results, including the report(s) of the other physician(s) consulted, must regularly be noted in the patient's medical record.

By comparison, the Dutch Act is very brief. Section 2.1 (a-d) stipulates that the physician must be convinced that there was a voluntary and well-considered request by the patient, that there was hopeless and unbearable suffering on the part of the patient, he must have informed the patient about the situation and about his prospects, and must have come to the conclusion, with the patient, that for the particular situation there was no other reasonable solution. Subsection (e) of the same section stipulates that the physician must consult at least one other independent physician who must see the patient and make a written assessment of the due care requirements indicated in sub-sections (a) through (d). All these requirements must however be supplemented with the requirements of good medical practice as established by reports and documents from medical and other organizations. Thus, the physician should discuss the matter with the patient's direct family and friends (unless the patient does not desire this, or there exist other good reasons for not doing so), and with the nursing personnel who are in direct contact with the requesting patient.[31] The physician must also maintain a complete medical record that includes details about how he has complied with the legal requirements.

In general, it seems to be a reasonable conclusion that the differences between the Belgian and Dutch Acts regarding this point are, from a material point of view, minor. The important difference lies in the additional requirements imposed by the Belgian Act in the case of a non-terminal patient. From a more formal point of view, on the other hand, the differences are indeed of some importance. In the introduction we noted that, in principle, only the legislative requirements are relevant as far as criminal law in the Netherlands is concerned. All additional criteria are primarily, though not exclusively, of importance in disciplinary proceedings. In the Belgian Act, the legislative criteria are, of course, also potentially relevant in criminal proceedings, but these legislative criteria are extremely detailed, unlike the terms of the Dutch Act. One possible explanation for this difference is that Belgian medical disciplinary law differs markedly from its Dutch counterpart. In Belgium the aim is primarily to maintain the honour and dignity of the profession. In practice this means

---

[31] J. Griffiths, A. Bood & H. Weyers, *Euthanasia and Law in the Netherlands*, p. 106.

that the disciplinary judge generally does not hear cases, as in the
Netherlands, dealing with the professional behaviour of physicians
towards their patients, but is more active in the area of behaviour
among colleagues. Another explanation might be that, in Belgium, the
political debate on euthanasia was not legally pre-structured: there
existed no precedents on this issue (as in the Netherlands), and the
parliamentary debates had to start from zero. Consequently, the complete results of the debates can be found in the Act, since it is the Act,
and the Act only, that provides legal norms. In the Netherlands the
case law on this issue is still relevant. Finally, there is also the possibility that the Belgian legislature did not have a great deal of confidence in the willingness of the Belgian Order of Physicians — which
is the main association of physicians in Belgium, and an organization
comparable to the General Medical Council in the United Kingdom
— to support the practice of euthanasia in a constructive manner. As
far as this is concerned, in the Netherlands, the Royal Dutch Medical
Association was in the 1970s and 1980s quick to propagate physicians' openness to euthanasia, which meant that the judiciary was
given the opportunity to play a more formative role in the process of
creating case law. The Belgian Order of Physicians has however not
shown much willingness to influence the political legislative process.
The Order was of the opinion that it would be better if the euthanasia question were left entirely up to the profession itself. In the spring
of 2000, during the hearings on the Euthanasia Act in the Belgian
Senate, the Order's vice-president stated that

> the National Council [of the Belgian Order of Physicians] does not
> wish to pass judgement either for or against any legislative initia-
> tives in this matter. (...) Nevertheless, a pressing question in our
> minds is whether a legislative initiative will bring us greater legal
> certainty. Of course it will, some say, because everything will be
> established in an act. We, the physicians and lawyers of the National
> Council, are however not so certain that legal certainty will thereby
> be assured. (...) There is also the question of whether the doctor-
> patient relationship, to which we attach supreme importance, will
> not be undermined by the new connotation introduced of the doc-
> tor as a bringer of death. As physicians, we feel very uncomfortable
> in such a role, perhaps because we are not yet used to such a role,
> but that does nothing to diminish our unease.

In short, whereas the Royal Dutch Medical Association — together
with the judiciary — played quite an important role in the Dutch

legislative process, the same can certainly not be said of the Belgian Order of Physicians. The Belgian Order has not been advocating for legislation, to say the least, and adopted an attitude of extreme reticence.

5.2. *The advance directive*

Due to the fact that the Belgian Act, as we saw above, contains specific provisions in cases where the request is formulated by means of an advance directive, there are also specific provisions with respect to the physician. Broadly speaking, they are the same requirements that are imposed on the physician when confronted with a conscious patient who requests euthanasia.

6. The Reporting Procedure

How can one encourage physicians to subject the practice of euthanasia to external supervision and control? This is the task inevitably facing any government that comes to the conclusion that traditional means of protecting life via a strict criminal prohibition of euthanasia does not in fact fulfil what it promises. Therefore, moving on from legislation regulating euthanasia, commissions have been created in the Netherlands and Belgium whose task it is to supervise the Euthanasia Act. In a sense, these commissions assume the role of what should normally be done by the public prosecutor. As a result, what had previously been an exclusively criminal assessment has been modified to become a more professionally and socially oriented assessment, with the criminal law more in the background. The aim of this is encourage physicians — who are understandably wary of the criminal justice system — to report their actions. This will yield better insight into the actual practice of euthanasia, thus leading to better social control and hopefully improvements in the practice.

Therefore, section 5 of the Belgian Act stipulates that a physician who has performed euthanasia must complete a registration document[32] and submit it within four working days of the euthanasia

---

[32] The document can be found in French at *www.health.fgov.be/AGP/fr/euthanasie/index.htm.*

being performed to the 'Federal Control and Evaluation Commission' established by the Act. By virtue of section 8 of the Act, the commission must study the completed registration document, which consists of a non-anonymous and an anonymous part, and determine on the basis of the anonymous section of the registration document whether or not the euthanasia was performed in accordance with the conditions and procedures provided for in the Act. The commission — which is composed of 16 members (eight physicians, four lawyers and four members 'from groups charged with the problem of incurably ill patients') — can, in cases of doubt, decide by simple majority to suspend anonymity. The commission must then inspect the non-anonymous section of the registration document. The commission may request from the attending physician any part of the patient's medical record that concerns the euthanasia. During the parliamentary debates, however, it became apparent that the physician might refuse to provide such information on the basis of professional confidentiality, though of course the physician would then be regarded with suspicion. This point raises the question of the extent of the *nemo tenetur* principle. Although it is not clear how far the right not to incriminate oneself extends — does it also apply to a *potential* suspect such as a physician who performs euthanasia? — this construction creates some tension with the *nemo tenetur* principle. The commission must pronounce judgement on the matter within two months. If the commission holds, in a decision taken by a two-thirds majority, that the conditions provided for in the Act have not been fulfilled, then it must refer the dossier to the public prosecutor of the jurisdiction in which the patient died.

The Dutch Act established so-called regional assessment commissions, of which five are currently functioning.[33] They were set up in 1998 and comprise three members each (and three substitutes): a physician, an expert in ethical questions, and a lawyer, the latter acting as chair. If euthanasia is performed, the physician in question submits a report to the assessment commission in his region. This commission is tasked with assessing compliance with the due care requirements as provided for in the Dutch Act. The commission's well-founded judgement, taken by simple majority vote, must be

---

[33] For an overview of the experiences of physician's with a regional commission, see the contribution of M. VAN DIJK, G.A.M. WIDDERSHOVEN & A.M. MEERSHOEK in this volume, pp. 71-82.

communicated to the physician within six weeks. Either the commission or the physician may request the judgement to be clarified. In the event of a negative judgement, the commission must notify the public prosecutor as well as the regional health inspectorate.

There are a number of striking similarities between the Belgian and Dutch Acts on this aspect. For instance, in both systems reporting is a necessary condition for legitimacy, and only suspicious cases are referred to the public prosecutor. In both systems, the reporting commissions function as a kind of buffer between physician and prosecutor, based on the idea that a physician does not want to be dealt with in an atmosphere of criminality. The intention, of course, is to make the reporting rate as optimal as possible. Finally, in both systems the public prosecutor's office is still empowered to launch an independent investigation, in accordance with that authority's autonomy.

There are, however, also a number of striking differences. The Dutch reporting procedure builds on the physician's duty to report deaths, which existed long before there was any talk of regulating euthanasia.[34] A similar duty to report deaths has never existed in Belgium. Indeed, Belgium is notorious for the high number of exhumations that take place, probably due to the lack of an efficient system for registering deaths. Moreover, whereas it is accepted in the Netherlands that euthanasia is not a natural death, in Belgium the debate on this matter has only just begun. In any event, the Act itself has not done anything to clarify this point. Section 15 of the Belgian Euthanasia Act states that a person who dies as a result of euthanasia performed in accordance with the conditions established by the Act, is *deemed* to have died a natural death for the purposes of the execution of any contracts to which he was party, in particular insurance contracts. One might conclude from this that euthanasia as such brings about an unnatural death.

Finally, the administrative organization of the Belgian federal commission is not without problems. Can a commission composed of 16 non-fulltime members possibly give serious consideration to all the files, especially now that there will be hundreds, if not thousands

---

[34] J. GRIFFITHS, 'Self-regulation by the Dutch medical profession that potentially shortens life' in H. KRABBENDAM & H.-M. TEN NAPEL (eds.), *Regulating Morality: A comparison of the role of the state in mastering the mores in the Netherlands and the United States*, Antwerp, Maklu, 2000, pp. 173-190.

per year? At the very least, there will need to be extensive administrative support and assistance.

7. Conclusion

Belgium and the Netherlands are at this moment the only two countries in the world that have legislation concerning euthanasia.[35] In this article we attempted a comparison between both Acts, with a focus on the Belgian Act. Although it seems fair to conclude that, from an *ethical* point of view, the general outlook of both Acts is rather liberal, there are also striking differences between them. For example, the exclusion of assisted suicide in the Belgian Act; the procedural steps that have to be followed by physician and patient before euthanasia can be legitimately performed; the status of the advance directive; as well as the possibility to refuse a medically meaningful alternative treatment. More generally, the Dutch Act is more concise than the Belgian Act. This is due to the fact that in the Netherlands before April 2002, when the Dutch Act came into effect, there existed a long established and legally accepted practice concerning euthanasia (and assisted suicide). As a consequence, legal certainty is also attained by, for example, established case law and guidelines of due care. In Belgium, case law was, and still is, nonexistent. As a result, the Belgian legislature has opted for a detailed and extensive regulation in order to achieve the maximum legal certainty for physician and patient. As we have seen, it is questionable whether the Belgian Parliament has succeeded in this, since many aspects of the Act still remain unclear.

References

ADAMS, M., 'Euthanasia: the Process of Legal Change in Belgium. Reflections on the Parliamentary Debate' in A. KLIJN, M. OTLOWSKI &

---

[35] Note that assisted suicide is legalized in the U.S. State of Oregon, since the Oregon Death with Dignity Act allows terminally ill Oregon residents to obtain, from their physicians, prescriptions for lethal medications for self-administration. The Act specifically prohibits euthanasia, where a physician or other person directly administers a medication to end another's life.

M. TRAPPENBURG (eds.), *Regulating Physician-Negotiated Death*, The Hague, Elsevier, 2001, pp. 29-47.

DELIENS, L., F. MORTIER, J. BILSEN, M. COSYNS, R. VANDER STICHELE, J. VANOVERLOOP & K. INGELS, 'End-of-life Decisions in Medical Practice in Flanders, Belgium' in *The Lancet* 356(2000), pp. 1806-1811.

GEVERS, J. & J. LEGEMAATE, 'Physician assisted suicide in psychiatry: an analysis of case law and professional options' in D.C. THOMASMA, T. KIMBROUGH KUSHNER, G.K. KIMSMA & C. CIESIELSKI-CARLUCCI (eds.), *Asking to die. Inside the Dutch debate about euthanasia*, Dordrecht, Kluwer Academic Publishers, 1997, pp. 71-91.

GRIFFITHS, J., A. BOOD & H. WEYERS, *Euthanasia and Law in the Netherlands*, Amsterdam, Amsterdam University Press, 1998.

GRIFFITHS, J., 'Self-regulation by the Dutch medical profession that potentially shortens life' in H. KRABBENDAM & H.-M. TEN NAPEL (eds.), *Regulating Morality: A comparison of the role of the state in mastering the mores in the Netherlands and the United States*, Antwerp, Maklu, 2000, pp. 173-190.

GRIFFITHS, J. & A. KLIJN, 'Can doctors' hands be bound? Advance directives under current Dutch law', 1999. To be found at *http://ww.rechten.rug.nl/mbpsl/milaanpa.htm*.

JANS, J., 'Euthanasiegesetzgebung in Belgien. Eine Übersicht über die politisch-ethische Debatte 1997-1999' in A. BONDOLFI & S. GROTENFELD (eds.), *Ethik und Gesetzgebung. Probleme — Lösungsversuche — Konzepte*, Stuttgart, Verlag W.Kolhammer, 2000, pp. 175-187.

NYS, H., 'Advice of the Federal Advisory Committee on Bioethics concerning legalization of euthanasia' in *European Journal of Health Law* 4(1997), pp. 389-393.

LEENEN, H.J.J., 'The development of euthanasia in the Netherlands' in *European Journal of Health Law* 8(2001), pp.125-133.

WEYERS, H., 'Euthanasia: the Process of Legal Change in The Netherlands. The Making of Requirements of Careful Practice' in A. KLIJN, M. OTLOWSKI & M. TRAPPENBURG (eds.), *Regulating Physician-Negotiated Death*, The Hague, Elsevier, 2001, pp. 1-27.

WILLIAMS, G., *The Sanctity of Life and the Criminal Law*, New York, Knopf, 1957.

PALLIATIVE CARE AND EUTHANASIA
BELGIAN AND DUTCH PERSPECTIVES

Bert Broeckaert & Rien Janssens

Introduction

Within a period of one year, two countries have enacted laws that articulate conditions under which euthanasia and physician assisted suicide (PAS) are permitted. Belgium and the Netherlands thus distinguish themselves from all other countries of the world.

In Belgium, palliative care organisations have been pro-actively involved in the debate, highlighting that if euthanasia can ever be justified, it is necessary to provide good palliative care for all by including in the Euthanasia Act a so-called 'palliative filter', *i.e.* a compulsory prior consultation with a specialised palliative care team. In the Netherlands, before the Euthanasia Act was enacted, there had been a policy of pragmatic tolerance for decades. The enactment itself did not give rise to intense debate. It can be questioned whether the new law would change anything at all since it only officially sanctioned an existing practice. This however does not mean that caregivers in palliative care, together with palliative care organisations, have not participated in the euthanasia debate.

In the first part of this article the input of palliative care organisations in the Dutch euthanasia debate is described and explained. First, opinions on euthanasia of a variety of palliative care organisations are described. Secondly, the Dutch debate on palliative care and euthanasia is analysed and evaluated. A brief introduction to Belgian palliative care is given followed by an overview of how palliative care organisations have participated in the Belgian euthanasia debate. Special attention will be given to the discussion on palliative sedation, sedation being presented by some as the palliative alternative to euthanasia but seen by others as nothing but euthanasia in disguise.

1. Dutch Organised Palliative Care's Views on Euthanasia

Let us start our discussion in the Netherlands and have a brief look at the attitude taken by Dutch organised palliative care towards euthanasia and the recent Euthanasia Act. The position of the national palliative care network organisation 'the Netherlands Palliative Care Network for Terminally Ill Patients' (NPTN, 'Netwerk Palliatieve Zorg voor Terminale Patiënten Nederland') is clear. Because it wants to respect the pluralism in Dutch society, it does not take a stance towards euthanasia and PAS. The organisation of palliative care in the Netherlands is characterised by a large number of nursing homes. 'Arcares', the national association for nursing homes and homes for the elderly, takes the same neutral stance towards euthanasia.

The Dutch hospices vary to a large extent as far as their attitude towards euthanasia is concerned. Most of these hospices are run by volunteers who also visit the patients in their own homes. They are called low-care hospices but many prefer the term 'almost-at-home-homes' ('bijna thuishuizen'). The general practitioner of the patients remains responsible for the medical care. Up until 2001, many of these hospices were members of the association 'Dutch Hospice Movement' (NHB, 'Nederlandse Hospice Beweging'). In that year, the NHB was succeeded by the association 'Volunteers Hospice Care in the Netherlands' (VHN, 'Vrijwilligers Hospicezorg Nederland'). It has never taken a stance for or against euthanasia. Euthanasia is considered to be a matter between the general practitioner and the patient. If houses wanted to become a member of the NHB, they were not allowed to base themselves on a religious conviction and take an official stance against euthanasia and PAS. The same view has been adopted by the VHN. There are also a small number of almost-at-home-homes with a Christian foundation (that are not members of the NHB). Their aims resemble those of the other homes but inside these hospices, euthanasia is not provided.

Apart from the almost-at-home-homes associated with the VHN and a small number of Christian houses, there are 15 so-called high-care hospices in the Netherlands. These hospices have a physician specialised in palliative care. Regular consultations are provided to general practitioners who take care of patients in their homes and to medical specialists in hospital wards. Fourteen out of these 15 high-care hospices are Christian even though patients are never refused because of their religious background. Within these hospices, euthanasia is not considered an option. If patients persist in their request they can be referred to their general practitioner or a medical specialist. Since the vast majority of the Dutch physicians and of the Dutch population in general do under certain conditions agree to euthanasia, they can be seen as a critical minority. All hospices want to show that through compassionate care, many euthanasia requests can be prevented or taken away.[1] Hospice physicians realise that their negative stance towards euthanasia makes them vulnerable to critique from outside. In a recently published book on palliative care in the Netherlands, a hospice physician is quoted as saying: "this is food for critics. But still I would not want it any other way. Moving a patient on his last day is not pleasant. But if I would have euthanasia carried out here, it would be dangerous for the future of the hospice. People should feel secure in this house, and if they would know that euthanasia would be carried out here, the safety and the clarity would vanish. Without that clarity I would not be able to work here."[2] Another hospice physician states: "Absolutely, there is a direct connection between the quality of palliative care and the demand for euthanasia. The demand decreases if the quality of care increases. But there will always be a group of people that persists in their request for euthanasia. Whatever you offer."[3] It is generally acknowledged that good palliative care cannot prevent or take away all requests for euthanasia.

It can be concluded that national organisations for palliative care consider euthanasia to be a matter between physician and patient. They do not take a stance towards euthanasia. Especially the individual high-care hospices however, have not stopped to stress that euthanasia cannot be justified if good palliative care for all is not or insufficiently available.

Yet, principal statements against euthanasia do not get much public support. The liberal climate in the Netherlands has contributed to the idea that euthanasia, though in need of political and legal regulation and control, is principally a matter between physician and

---

[1] R. JANSSENS, H. TEN HAVE & Z. ZYLICZ, 'Hospice and euthanasia in the Netherlands. An ethical point of view' in *Journal of Medical Ethics* 25(1999), pp. 408-412.

[2] R. BRUNTINK, *Een goede plek om te sterven. Palliatieve zorg in Nederland. Een wegwijzer* [A good place to die. Palliative care in the Netherlands. A guide], Zutphen, Plataan, 2002.

[3] *Ibid.*

patient. However, as will be indicated below, in spite of the liberal climate and the respect for ethical pluralism, recent developments in palliative care have had a substantial impact on the Dutch euthanasia debate.

2. Palliative Care and Euthanasia. The Dutch Debate

In the context of the European 'Pallium' project on palliative care, a questionnaire on ethical issues in palliative care was sent in 1999 to 2 200 European caregivers involved in palliative care. It came as no surprise that of the 768 repondents, only 41 (*i.e.* 5,3 percent) could conceive of extreme situations in which euthanasia could be a part of palliative care. No less than 89,2 percent of the respondents rejected euthanasia.[4] Remarkably, a comparison of these figures with the large scale research study that was conducted in the Netherlands in 2001 reveals opposite figures. Eighty-nine percent of Dutch physicians involved in end-of-life care can conceive of situations in which euthanasia and physician assisted suicide are justifiable and 57 percent have actually carried out euthanasia or physician assisted suicide. Ten percent would not carry out euthanasia but would refer patients to obtain euthanasia from a colleague. Only 1 percent reject euthanasia and physician assisted suicide and would not refer patients.[5]

From abroad, reproaches have been made that the Netherlands has insufficient palliative care and would thus need the option of euthanasia and PAS. Or it was stated that the many cases of euthanasia and PAS (3 800 cases in 2001) could explain the absence of palliative care since Dutch physicians always had an 'easy way out'. Dutch physicians and ethicists attending international congresses had to defend themselves in front of a homogeneous audience. Only few attended.[6]

Fortunately, the times have changed. When the Minister of Health wrote in 1996 in a letter to the Dutch Parliament that palliative care

---

[4] R. JANSSENS *et al.*, 'Palliative care in Europe. Towards a more comprehensive understanding' in *European Journal of Palliative Care* 8(2001), pp.20-23.

[5] G. VAN DER WAL & P.J. VAN DER MAAS, *Euthanasie en andere medische beslissingen rond het levenseinde* [Euthanasia and other medical decisions at the end of life], Den Haag, Sdu, 1996.

[6] Z. ZYLICZ, 'Hospice in Holland. The story behind the blank spot' in *American Journal of Hospice and Palliative Care* 4(1993), pp. 30-34.

was to be further developed, it was also an answer to the reproaches from abroad.[7] And it was this letter that marked the beginnings of increasing government support for palliative care. Plans are now being made to develop about 70 to 80 local networks in which the different palliative care settings cooperate. Regionally, specialist palliative care centres will be attached to the Integral Cancer Centres and/or the academic hospitals. Nationally, the NPTN will continue its function as network organisation.[8] The reproaches from abroad about the *relative* underdevelopment of palliative care remain difficult if not impossible to prove. One of the most significant successes of the Dutch palliative care community is the organisation of the EAPC congress (the congress of the European Association for Palliative Care) in The Hague in 2003. This indicates that opinions from abroad have become better informed and more sensitised. International cooperation is now developing.

These important developments in palliative care together with a burgeoning sensitisation of the international views on euthanasia and palliative care in the Netherlands do not mean that there are no problems to be dealt with — on the contrary. Precisely because palliative care has only recently become the focus of attention, relatively little attention has thus far been paid to the prevention of requests for euthanasia. The debate in the Netherlands has focused on data, procedures and assessment of the requirements under which euthanasia would be tolerable. The implicit — and problematic — idea has been that when patients request euthanasia, they want (a) to die and (b) to have their lives actively terminated.[9] These assumptions are now increasingly under debate.

Very revealing was a newspaper article with the title 'Remorse. Proponents of euthanasia reorient themselves' that appeared in November 2001.[10] It was an interview with SCEA physicians (SCEN

---

[7] DEPARTMENT OF HEALTH, WELFARE AND SPORTS, *Palliatieve zorg in de terminale fase* [Palliative care in the terminal phase], Letter to the Chairman of the House of Representatives of the States General, 18 April 1996.

[8] DEPARTMENT OF HEALTH, WELFARE AND SPORTS, *Definitief standpunt palliatieve zorg* [Final position on palliative care], Letter to the Chairman of the House of Representatives of the States General, 11 March 2002.

[9] R. JANSSENS, *Palliative care. Concepts and ethics*, Nijmegen, Nijmegen University Press, 2001.

[10] M. OOSTVEEN, 'Spijt. Voorvechters van de euthanasiepraktijk bezinnen zich [Remorse. Proponents of euthanasia reorient themselves]' in *NRC Handelsblad*, 10 November 2001.

physicians in Amsterdam). In order to safeguard the requirements of the Dutch euthanasia regulation, all over the country a number of physicians are educated to provide adequate support and consultation to physicians who consider carrying out euthanasia. These physicians are called SCEN physicians (Support and Consultation in Case of Euthanasia in the Netherlands, 'Steun en Consultatie bij Euthanasie in Nederland').

Most of the SCEA physicians ('Support and Consultation in Case of Euthanasia in Amsterdam') in the article were used to serve about 15 to 20 times a year as consultant for colleagues considering carrying out euthanasia. However, those who have received education in palliative care now state that they have started at the wrong side. They realise that people have been directed into a euthanasia procedure while much could still be done about the quality of life. Whilst they were focused on euthanasia, they lost sight of alternative measures. Having been educated in palliative care, the focus is now on the requirement that euthanasia can only be justified if no alternative measures are viable. Without knowledge of these measures, it is impossible to assess the unbearability and hopelessness of suffering. With the knowledge of today, many cases of euthanasia of the past would have been prevented. One physician stated that since she no longer brings up euthanasia herself, the requests of patients also disappear. Many patients, not all, are comfortable with the offer of good palliative care. On the other hand it is stated that exactly because of the new law, some patients now consider euthanasia a right. Patients do not request euthanasia anymore, they demand it. But due to the developments in palliative care, the interviewed physicians now have the confidence to reject requests if they are not convinced of the unbearability and hopelessness of the suffering or if alternative measures are available.

Regarding this newspaper article, a reaction from the Minister of Health was requested by the Christian parties and the Socialist Party in the Dutch Parliament. In her reaction, the minister informed the Parliament that she agreed to the message of the SCEA physicians and that restraint with regard to life-terminating acts has always been the intention of the cabinet.[11] She admitted that, due to the

---

[11] HOUSE OF REPRESENTATIVES OF THE STATES GENERAL, *Toetsing van levensbeëindiging op verzoek en hulp bij zelfdoding en wijziging van het Wetboek van Strafrecht en van de Wet op de Lijkbezorging (26 691)* [Review of life termination and assisted suicide and

recent developments in palliative care, alternative measures have become available whereas some years ago, without the knowledge of today, physicians were more inclined to carry out the patient's request for euthanasia. But, in the view of the minister, palliative care and euthanasia principally remain connected since even the best palliative care cannot always relieve suffering to a tolerable degree. Euthanasia can be a worthy end of a disease process in which good palliative care was provided. The painful truth remains that lives have been terminated because of inadequate knowledge of palliative care. And since palliative care is still developing it is safe to state that this problematic practice has not yet been abolished.

In some cases patients really want to die since they cannot bear their hopeless suffering anymore. Regarding these patients, the subject of sedation at the end of life is now getting attention. Very little is known about the practice of sedation in the Netherlands.[12] The ethical debate has mainly been held abroad since the implicit assumption in the Netherlands has been that patients who request euthanasia want to have their lives actively terminated. Yet, more voices in Dutch society are now questioning this assumption. Can sedation be a viable alternative to euthanasia? In the context of this article, let it suffice to note that when, apart from euthanasia, the subject of sedation is also discussed, patients are presented with the possibility of more than one option. They are given a choice. It may well appear that some patients may prefer not to be killed by the physician who has cared for them. Sedation may be a preferable option for them. Others may stick with their request to have their lives actively ended. These are difficult cases in which, as was already indicated above, the autonomous requests of the patient can never be the only argument.[13] Concludingly, because palliative care is now under development, the euthanasia debate in the Netherlands is widening. Alternative palliative measures are stressed and many physicians do carefully assess what patients really mean when they request

amendment of the criminal code and the burial and cremation act], Letter of the Minister of Health, Welfare and Sports, no. 44, 22 November 2001.

[12] R. JANSSENS et al., 'Controversen rondom terminale sedatie [Controversies on terminal sedation]' in Tijdschrift voor Geneeskunde en Ethiek 12(2002), pp. 79-83.

[13] A large scale empirical and ethical study on the issue of sedation at the end of life is currently being conducted at the University Medical Center of Nijmegen, in close cooperation with Catholic University of Leuven. See R. JANSSENS et al., 'The ethics of decision-making when suffering has become refractory. The case of Belgium

euthanasia. At the same time, much more can and must be done. Education in palliative care is still not part of many medical curricula. The law does not obligate physicians who consider carrying out euthanasia to consult a SCEN physician (whose responsibility it is to assess possible palliative alternatives) or a specialist in palliative care. The number of specialists is low. Much can be done to improve consultations before active life-terminating acts are carried out. And as more and more physicians are getting convinced that careful assessment of the nature and causes of suffering of the patient, together with knowledge and expertise in palliative care, can prevent or take away many euthanasia requests, one of the challenges for the future is to create better possibilities for careful *a priori* consultation.[14]

3. Palliative Care in Belgium

Unlike the Netherlands, Belgium was, at least until very recently, as far as euthanasia is concerned, a very ordinary country. But in May 2002, Belgium became the second country in the world to have a Euthanasia Act.[15] Before we concentrate on the way organised palliative care has reacted to this sudden development, we thought it would be wise to write a few lines on palliative care in Belgium. Though fairly young, palliative care in Belgium developed rapidly. Due to a very fruitful cooperation between palliative care and the Belgian authorities, nationwide a unique and comprehensive legal and organisational palliative care framework was set up. This happened only very recently, in the second half of the previous decade. In order to organise palliative care nationwide the Belgian territory has been divided into about 30 regions. In each region a so-called palliative network or local palliative care cooperative is responsible for the coordination of palliative care. Linked to each network is a palliative support team that gives palliative support to general home

---

and the Netherlands' in *Abstracts of the 8th congress of the European Association for Palliative Care*, 2-5 April 2003, The Hague, the Netherlands, p. 94.

[14] H. TEN HAVE & R. JANSSENS, 'Toetsing van euthanasie. Verbetering terminale zorg noodzakelijk [Review of euthanasia. Optimisation of terminal care is necessary]' in *Christen Democratische Verkenningen* 5(1997), pp.186-193.

[15] See also B. BROECKAERT, 'Belgium: Towards a legal recognition of euthanasia' in *European Journal of Health Law* 8(2001), pp. 95-107.

care. There are other palliative support teams as well, for in accordance with the law, every single hospital and recognised nursing home is to have a palliative support team of its own. Finally a small number of palliative care units are available in each region.[16]

Characteristic of the way palliative care is thus organised is that Belgium has opted for multi-layered palliative care, starting with palliative support teams at home, support teams in hospitals and nursing homes and finishing with palliative care units. Palliative home care that enables terminally ill patients to die at home (something most terminally ill patients would prefer) is thus seen as the first and basic layer of palliative care. A second characteristic is that palliative care is intended to be fully integrated in general health care, hence the stress on the supportive and educational mission of specialised palliative care services. We do not want to suggest that Belgium is a palliative care paradise. The framework that has been developed is indeed quite unique and very good, but its implementation started only a few years ago. Some serious financial problems remain and in any case, the large amount of good work being done by those people who are active in palliative care does not alter the fact that there are still too many people who are not reached by them, that there are still too many patients who reach the final phase of their illness without adequate palliative care.

4. A palliative care reaction

With *Palliative Care, Euthanasia and Dying with Dignity*, a text that was published in January 2000, the 'Federation Palliative Care Flanders' (FPZV, 'Federatie Palliatieve Zorg Vlaanderen') — the organisation that unites all Flemish palliative care services in the Dutch-speaking part of Belgium — did not intend to present a comprehensive standpoint regarding euthanasia or the bill on euthanasia that was submitted on 20 December 1999.[17] Being a pluralistic

---

[16] For an introduction to Belgian palliative care, see B. BROECKAERT, 'Le cure palliative in Belgio [Palliative care in Belgium]' in *Bioetica e Cultura* 8(1999), pp. 45-54; B. BROECKAERT & P. SCHOTSMANS, 'Palliative Care in Belgium', in H. TEN HAVE & R. JANSSENS (eds.), *Palliative Care in Europe. Concepts and Policies*, Amsterdam, IOS Press — Ohmsha, 2001, pp. 31-42.

[17] FEDERATION PALLIATIVE CARE FLANDERS, *Palliatieve zorg, euthanasie en menswaardig sterven* [Palliative care, euthanasia and dying with dignity], Position statement in response to the bills on euthanasia and palliative care submitted on 29 December, Wemmel, 27 January 2000.

organisation at the service of all terminally ill persons, the FPZV stated it could not and should not do this. Instead the FPZV wanted to focus only on the way the relation between euthanasia and palliative care was presented in the bill on euthanasia. By high-lighting four basic but problematic assumptions of the December 1999 bill (and of a lot of other bills on euthanasia) and by making some important suggestions it tried to show where from a palliative care point of view the real and big problems lie and what could be done about them.

The bills concerning the end of life submitted by the governing parties on 20 December 1999 had the merit of not being exclusively focused on euthanasia. In addition to two bills on euthanasia, a third bill was submitted that concerned palliative care. Though it was for-mulated in vague and general terms, this proposal explicitly stated that every patient suffering from an incurable illness has the right to palliative care. A federal plan drafted by the minister of Social Affairs and Public Health must ensure that this right is not neglected. There must be broad, accessible, and high-quality care to respond to the rights of the individual patient. It is self-evident that the Flemish Pal-liative Care Federation fully supported this exceptionally ambitious, but at the same time medically, socially and ethically necessary goal. Anyone suffering from an incurable illness, however, derives little benefit from overblown declarations; what they need is effective care. The FPZV therefore said it hoped and expected that in the short term the government would make every necessary effort — in the first place budgetary — to promote the further expansion of high-quality palliative care. The FPZV also stated it hoped and expected that, just as in the past, an appeal would be made to the available expertise in the palliative care sector, and that in improving and expanding the supply of palliative care, the starting point would be thorough con-sultations between the palliative care sector and the responsible authorities.

5. Palliative Care and Euthanasia: One Correct and Three Incorrect Assumptions

It was of course no coincidence that the bill on palliative care was submitted at the same time as the bill on euthanasia. The bill on palliative care was linked with the one on euthanasia because the submitters were at pains to avoid that shortcomings in the system of palliative care might lead people to opt for euthanasia, for improper reasons and sometimes even against their will and beliefs. In such cases, it would be impossible to speak of freedom of choice regarding the end of life, which was one of the aims of the bills. In the absence of good palliative care, all that remains is the pseudo-choice between euthanasia and an intolerable, inhumane dying. This was the reason for having bills concerning euthanasia as well as a bill concerning palliative care.

Could anyone object to the juxtaposition of euthanasia and palliative care in the bills of 20 December 1999? In any case, the submitters were absolutely right in assuming that a legalization of euthanasia without a corresponding expansion of palliative care would have unacceptable consequences. The FPZV said it believed it was a good thing, then, that palliative care, also because of the necessary clarification of the euthanasia demand, received the required attention in a separate bill. However, can palliative care and euthanasia simply be placed next to each other, as if they were two completely separate alternatives? And was it advisable, except for one brief allusion (in article 3, cfr. infra), to not even mention palliative care in the bill on euthanasia? According to the FPZV the bill made four assumptions, three of which the Federation considered to be incorrect on the basis of its palliative expertise.

5.1. *First assumption: Some people die an inhumane death*

According to the FPZV it could not be denied that the submitters of the bills on euthanasia of 20 December 1899 made these joint proposals out of ethical considerations and a genuine concern for the fate of those who die in inhumane circumstances. And unfortunately the submitters were not mistaken when they assumed that there still are people who are confronted, on their deathbed, with "sustained and intolerable pain and distress". The FPZV did not contest the accuracy of this assumption made by the euthanasia proposals. Although healthcare in general has undoubtedly made great progress in this area, such dramatic and tragic experiences of dying are still an especially sad reality. Any family member, friend, acquaintance or caregiver who has experienced such dying nearby or from afar can only say, "this cannot happen", "never again". From the point of view of such experiences, a positive attitude to euthanasia would seem to be self-evident.

5.2. *Second assumption: palliative care is helpless in such cases*

What is missing from this all-too-human and quite understandable line of reasoning — people (would otherwise) die an inhumane death, hence euthanasia — is not the (unfortunately correct) presupposition that a certain number of people die an inhumane death. According to the FPZV, two additional and incorrect presuppositions make this reasoning particularly problematic. The first one amounts to assuming that incurably ill patients sometimes end their lives in degrading circumstances because nothing else is possible, because medicine is powerless in some cases, because, in some cases, "sustained and intolerable pain and distress that cannot be alleviated", are simply an unavoidable part of dying. But it is not because some people undeniably die an inhumane death that it *has* to be like this.

It was the FPZV's impression that those who submitted the bill, and a considerable fraction of public opinion, seriously underestimated the possibilities offered by specialized and multidisciplinary palliative care. Even without euthanasia, it is, according to the FPZV, almost always possible to permit incurably ill patients to die a humane, dignified death. Pain and other symptoms (nausea, angst, restlessness, shortness of breath) can all be handled in an adequate manner by specialized palliative care teams. Pain, for instance, can be effectively treated in close to 95 percent of cases by administering the appropriate pain medication. In extreme cases, where it seems impossible to bring certain physical or mental symptoms under sufficient control using medication that leaves the patient fully conscious, palliative care offers the possibility, in consultation with the patient and the family, to administer what is called 'palliative sedation'. Palliative sedation is the deliberate, measured reduction of the patient's level of consciousness to a point where one or more of the unmanageable symptoms (one speaks of "refractory symptoms") are suppressed to a sufficient degree (cf. infra).

The FPZV concluded that the second assumption of the current bill amounts to a serious underestimation of the ability of a complete palliative care regime to free the incurably ill patient from the "sustained and intolerable pain or distress" of which, in the absence of this care, he is too often a victim. Palliative care can bring it about that the reasons for a great many euthanasia requests simply disappear. This is why it is so important to make sufficient room within the bills concerning euthanasia for a contribution on the part of palliative care.

5.3. *Third assumption: The palliative expertise of the average physician*

Some people (would otherwise) die an inhumane death, hence euthanasia? This line of reasoning rests, according to the FPZV, on yet another, equally questionable presupposition, namely the idea that people who die in an inhumane way do this only after their physicians and caregivers have provided all the palliative care possible so as to spare the patient this bitter end. It is a mistake to believe, however, that the average physician or hospital ward possesses the necessary expertise and means for providing state-of-the-art palliative care. Already at the level of pain control — and effective pain control is absolutely essential in palliative care — the average medical treatment of incurably ill patients often exhibits grave shortcomings. Palliative know-how and the culture of palliative care are not yet generally available.

Was it not, however, very easy for the submitters of the recent bills to rebut this criticism? They could well reply that the objection mentioned here is undoubtedly well grounded, but that it in no way applied to them or to their proposals. It is quite possible that a number of people assume that the average physician and nurse are well acquainted with palliative knowledge and culture, but the submitters of these bills could not be accused of sharing this incorrect assumption. This, they could say, is clear from their bill concerning palliative care: in the clarification of the bill, it is very clearly stated that end-of-life support is an essential but often neglected task; there is also a clear indication of the necessity of training and additional updating for physicians and nurses. So this bill clearly does not share the contested assumption, but works from the *reverse* assumption, *i.e.*, that the principles of palliative care are as yet insufficiently applied, an assumption that is shared by the FPZV.

Does this kind of hypothetical correction fully deal with the criticism of the FPZV? The FPZV did not think so. Granted, in the bill concerning palliative care, the submitters indeed assumed that there was room for improvement in physicians' and caregivers' palliative expertise. But the bill on euthanasia speaks an entirely different language. Here, no questions at all are posed about the palliative competence of the physician involved. In the governing parties' bill on euthanasia of 20 December 1999, palliative care was only mentioned in article 3, which establishes the procedural conditions that a physician must meet in order to be able to grant a euthanasia request. A first procedural condition is that the physician involved must fully inform the patient about all aspects of his state of health and about *the various existing possibilities for palliative care and their consequences* (our emphasis). Further procedural conditions concern the other physician who must be consulted, the pain or distress and the patient's request, and the discussion about the request, if the patient so desires, with the nursing team, family, or other persons of the patient's choosing.

What is important for the argument of the FPZV is that palliative care was not mentioned in these further procedural conditions, nor did it come up directly or indirectly in the other articles of the bill. This means that the submitters of the bill seem to assume that all possible alternatives to euthanasia have been sufficiently considered and exhausted when: a) a patient turns out to be incurably ill; b) the patient's intolerable pain or distress continues, despite the efforts of the physician involved; c) the physician (and he alone) judges that this pain or distress cannot be alleviated; d) the physician has fully informed the patient about what palliative care might still be able to provide. In this way, the physician is assigned an extremely heavy responsibility. Nowhere does the bill state that the physician ought to possess a specific expertise in the area of palliative care; nowhere does it consider further consultation about the palliative possibilities to be necessary. Although the bill on euthanasia does speak of a second physician, his assessment only concerns the incurable character of the illness, not the patient's request or the patient's pain or distress. Nor is any specific competence in palliative care expected from the second physician. Whereas the bill on palliative care clearly indicates that there is room for improvement in the average physician's palliative expertise, in the bill on euthanasia the consulting physician's palliative expertise seems to be beyond all doubt — incorrectly in the FPZV's opinion. This, according to the FPZV, is an obvious contradiction.

The FPZV concluded from this that the bill on euthanasia did indeed work on the basis of the problematic assumption that the average physician possesses the palliative expertise required to adequately combat pain and suffering, to judge when pain or distress cannot be alleviated, and to properly inform the patient about the various palliative options and their consequences. If this bill in its current form were to become law, the FPZV believed that a good number of patients, as well as their physicians, might incorrectly think that their pain and distress cannot be brought under control, and might decide to "choose" euthanasia. But was it not precisely these pseudo-choices — one could refer to the comments accompanying the bill on euthanasia and the bill on palliative care — that the submitters of the euthanasia bill wanted to avoid at all costs? This is why, according to the FPZV, palliative care must be granted a larger place in the current bill on euthanasia.

5.4. *Fourth assumption: The autonomy of the intolerably suffering patient*

There were still other reasons why the FPZV thought it was not advisable to place palliative care and euthanasia next to each other as two completely detached alternatives and then to leave palliative care practically unmentioned in the bill on euthanasia. A fourth — and once again questionable — assumption made by the bill has to do with the putative autonomy of the incurably ill and intolerably suffering patient. It goes without saying that an incurably ill patient who suffers from intolerable pain and sees no end to the pain will quickly be driven to opt for euthanasia. It is equally clear that in such a case one can hardly speak of an autonomous choice. The pressure exerted by the utterly degrading circumstances in which the patient finds himself is so great at that moment that the patient's own will and convictions scarcely have any influence. For this reason, the FPZV firmly believes that in this case the patient's choice cannot be between palliative care and euthanasia. Palliative care is not some exotic or esoteric therapy available to the incurably ill patient as one possible choice in addition to euthanasia. It is, or rather should be, an active and total approach with which medicine and healthcare respond to the patient's needs and, in this sense, it is more a self-evident point of departure than a conscious and explicit choice made by the patient.

If one really wants to respect the patient's autonomy and freedom of choice, then it is of the utmost importance that incurably ill patients are treated according to the principles of palliative care (care for their physical, mental, social and spiritual needs; interdisciplinary approach; active care; etc.). Only by ensuring this condition is met can one avoid that many people request and receive euthanasia for the wrong reasons — reasons having more to do with the shortcomings of our healthcare system than with the patient's autonomous

will. The submitters of the bill are right when they state that palliative care cannot resolve or prevent every request for euthanasia.
There will indeed always be people who continue to request
euthanasia, even with the best palliative measures in place, and even
when the physical and mental symptoms from which they suffer
have been brought under control. In many cases these are people
who want out because they consider their lives to be no longer meaningful, no longer worth the effort. It is on the basis of these considerations, the level of meaning, rather than the level of a purely physical or psychological problematic, that their request for euthanasia
should be understood. But everyday dealings with dying people has
taught the caregivers of the FPZV that only a very small minority of
patients who request euthanasia belong to this category. With the
vast majority of patients requesting euthanasia, the request vanishes
after they have encountered the beneficial effects produced by good
palliative care. Experience in dealing with the dying has shown that
the largest fraction of incurably ill patients do not want euthanasia;
they want to live, even in the final months, weeks and days. Palliative care is not so much about humane *dying*, but rather humane *living* in the face of death.

To conclude: just like the two previous, and equally contestable
assumptions of the current bill concerning euthanasia, this faulty
estimation of the suffering patient's autonomy also leaves the way
open for a number of choices for euthanasia which are not really
choices at all but rather should be understood as requests for help.
In light of the untenability of three of the four assumptions, it would,
according to the Flemish Palliative Care Federation, seem to be inad-
visable to juxtapose euthanasia and palliative care and present them
as two equally viable alternatives. Good palliative care can ensure
that only the genuine requests for euthanasia remain. What is
urgently needed then is more attention to palliative care, also in the
bill on euthanasia

6. Specific Proposals and Amendments

The January 2000 text of the FPZV not only discussed the relationship between palliative care and euthanasia in a rather general way,
it also included a number of specific proposals and amendments.
In order to respond to its fundamental points of criticism, for the

FPZV two things were essential, neither one of which could be ignored by politicians if they wanted to avoid euthanasia becoming a quick and convenient solution that shamelessly camouflages palliative incompetence. In the first place, the government must do everything possible to drastically increase the availability of good palliative care. For this reason, a further expansion of palliative care should be a top priority for both the federal and the Flemish governments. The FPZV stated it was absolutely unacceptable to wait until the end of 2001 before tabling a federal plan for palliative care. Something must be done in a very short period of time about the total lack of financing for palliative functions in rest and nursing homes, about the merely symbolic financing for palliative support teams in hospitals, and about the very low honoraria for physicians in palliative care units. Moreover, the palliative networks must be reinforced and palliative care and palliative medicine should acquire a significant place in a physician's and paramedic's education.

Secondly, precisely out of respect for the autonomy of incurably ill patients, the FPZV stated that it was necessary to alter the current bill on euthanasia at a number of points. Before a second physician is consulted (who, in the December 1999 proposal, would only assess the incurability of the illness), the FPZV thought it would be advisable: i) that the physician involved consult, on the basis of the patient's medical file, with the palliative support team of the own institution or the local palliative network concerning the concrete possibilities of palliative care for the patient in question; ii) that the palliative advice provided by the support team is communicated to the patient; and iii) that the patient is also explicitly given the opportunity to consult the palliative support team. The FPZV argued very clearly that it was not at all its intention to let the palliative support team decide about the patient's request for euthanasia — indeed, palliative care workers were not asking for this. It was its intention to ensure that the palliative possibilities are always made use of, or at least thoroughly discussed, so that euthanasia only occurs when the patient genuinely wants it. According to the FPZV it is simply not good enough when the physician involved (whose knowledge of and experience in palliative care in most cases would be very limited) is required to fully inform the patient about the various existing possibilities for palliative care and their consequences. To avoid pseudochoices a prior palliative consultation was absolutely necessary.

Palliative care and adequate treatment for incurably ill patients is not something that one does on one's own. A single physician, no matter how competent, cannot provide adequate palliative care. It is only by working as an interdisciplinary team that the active and integral care required by an incurably ill patient can be achieved. In light of this fundamental experience of palliative care, the FPZV thought it was absolutely necessary that the physician consult with the palliative support team about the various palliative possibilities. This is why the FPZV also thought it would be advisable — once again, in order to avoid pseudo-choices — that the role of the second physician be expanded in the bill on euthanasia. It would seem not unreasonable to ask that the second physician's advice also be obtained regarding the conditions imposed on the euthanasia request and regarding the question whether the patient's pain and distress is intolerable and inescapable. Two minds are always better than one, and in the case of such a delicate and irrevocable decision as granting a request for euthanasia, consultation and discussion are definitely suitable.

It is undeniable that paramedics and particularly nurses play a crucial role in the palliative team. Their everyday caring involvement with the dying patient teaches them a great deal about the patient's fears, questions and needs. They are in the best position to notice any small changes in the patient's condition which might have an enormous influence on the patient's quality of life. For this reason, the FPZV believed it to be self-evident that a physician should have prior consultation with the care team before granting any request for euthanasia. Finally, the FPZV thought it was also advisable that, in addition to the physician involved with the case, both the palliative care team and the second physician make their advice known to the federal evaluation commission for the law concerning euthanasia (or another supervisory body). If they also have these opinions at their disposal, the members of the commission would be better equipped to evaluate the law and to formulate recommendations.

7. A Palliative Filter in the Euthanasia Procedure

As far as the euthanasia discussion was concerned the Flemish Palliative Care Federation did not restrict itself to publishing the position paper we discussed so far. The ideas of the FPZV were spread through several interviews, opinions, articles, lectures and symposia. On the other hand a strong emphasis was laid on a constructive and open dialogue with the politicians involved in the euthanasia debate, especially those that had submitted the bill on euthanasia. There were several meetings with politicians, both at an individual and at a party level, resulting in regular contacts with the political world. During the euthanasia hearings in the commissions of the Belgian Senate and the House of Representatives palliative care and palliative care people got a lot of attention. Partly as a result of all these efforts and of the constructive and open attitude of the FPZV in general, the specific proposals and amendments of the FPZV were not disregarded.

The net result of the Belgian euthanasia debate and of the way palliative care had responded to it was a renewed interest in palliative care, a general awareness that the further development of palliative care was indeed absolutely essential. In 2001 the palliative care budget was doubled and adjusted precisely in the way Belgian organised palliative care had wanted it. The role of the 'second' physician was seriously expanded (though, of course, the FPZV had not been alone in its criticism on the minimal role played by this physician in the earlier bill). The FPZV was pleased with the fact that in the new bill, the present Euthanasia Act, the physician is required to consult with the nursing team (if present) before granting any request for euthanasia; however the FPZV was disappointed with the fact that its other and probably most important amendment regarding the involvement of the palliative support team in the euthanasia procedure was not present in the amended majority bill of March 2001. As a result of this in its later texts, written by Bert Broeckaert and published between September 2001 and May 2002, and in its contacts with the politicians in this period, the FPZV concentrated its efforts on getting support for this idea of a prior palliative consultation and on trying to have this compulsory consultation included in the euthanasia procedure.[18] Since the September 2001 text introduced the term 'palliative filter' to denote this idea of a prior palliative consultation

---

[18] See FEDERATION PALLIATIVE CARE FLANDEREN, *Federatie Palliatieve Zorg Vlaanderen pleit voor een palliatieve filter in de euthanasieprocedure* [Federation palliative care Flanders pleads for a palliative filter in the euthanasia procedure], Wemmel, 26 September 2001; B. BROECKAERT, W. DISTELMANS & A. MULLIE, *Nota aan de Voorzitters en Leden van de Commissie voor de Volksgezondheid en de Commissie voor de Justitie (Kamer van Volksvertegenwoordigers)* [Memorandum to the chairmen and members of the committees of public health and justice (Chamber of Representatives)], Wemmel,

intended to filter out pseudo-choices for euthanasia (the result of poor palliative care), this term became a rather popular and highly debated term in the Belgian euthanasia discussion.

Is it not enough to increase the availability of good palliative care? Why should one want to involve palliative care and the palliative support teams which, at least in Belgium, are available in each region (for home care) and in each hospital, in the euthanasia procedure? In the later texts of the FPZV seven reasons were given for doing so; reasons which only very briefly can be presented here.

1. A lot of euthanasia requests are in fact requests for help, camou-flaging a lack of adequate palliative care. When these people receive good palliative care, their quality of life improves drastically and as a consequence of this a lot of euthanasia requests simply disappear. Regarding this there is a very broad consensus among palliative care physicians, both in Belgium as internationally, whether they person-ally are religious or secular, in favour of or against euthanasia. There-fore, to avoid the numerous pseudo-choices for euthanasia that have to do with this lack of adequate palliative care, it is necessary to include in the euthanasia-procedure what one could call a palliative filter.

2. As a lot of physicians (and this is a well-known international prob-lem) do not possess the necessary palliative know-how and experi-ence, it is not unlikely at all that patients ask for euthanasia for the wrong reasons, that is lack of adequate care.

3. Even when physicians in general would know more about pallia-tive care then they do right now, this would not make them into pal-liative care specialists. Therefore when a physician is confronted with a request as delicate, radical and irreversible as a euthanasia request, it is only normal that a specialist is consulted, something that hap-pens a thousand time a day for problems often far less serious.

4. Starting from the notion of informed consent or informed request, one could say that an absolutely essential condition for euthanasia to be possibly acceptable is that there is an informed decision by both patient and physician. Now if one as a patient or as a physician does not know much about possible palliative alternatives — which often

7 January 2002; B. BROECKAERT, W. DISTELMANS & A. MULLIE, *Palliatieve zorg in de euthanasiewet. Open brief aan de Leden van de Kamer van Volksvertegenwoordigers* [Pallia-tive care in the euthanasia act. Open letter to the members of the Chamber of Repre-sentatives], Wemmel, 13 May 2002.

will be the case — an informed and therefore free and real choice for euthanasia is simply impossible. Because of the limited palliative expertise of the average physician, the principle of informed consent does not receive the respect it deserves, when, as in the present bill on euthanasia, one suggests that sufficient information on possible palliative alternatives is given when the attending physician, on the basis of his own very limited expertise, informs the patient "about the different existing possibilities of palliative care and their consequences" (art. 3).

5. If, as is often stipulated in euthanasia bills, euthanasia can only be permitted when no real alternatives are available, the only way one can make sure that in a particular case there are indeed no alternatives is, given the lack of palliative expertise of the average physician, by having the kind of palliative consultation the Flemish Palliative Care Federation is proposing.

6. By making it mandatory upon the physician to consult with the palliative support team, you overcome the ignorance and hesitation that often exists among physicians as far as palliative care and palliative services are concerned. Thus this compulsory consultation in an important way helps to further integrate palliative care in general health care. It is clear that this further integration would be a highly desirable side-effect of the FPZV proposal.

7. By offering physicians this palliative consultation you help them to make a sound decision. By making them feel confident about their decision, their compliance with the euthanasia procedure that has been developed is enhanced.

Taken together these seven arguments constitute a strong case in favour of including a palliative filter in the Euthanasia Act. But it is of course not enough to argue that a palliative support team should be involved in the euthanasia procedure. A central question to be answered here is how one actually sees and understands this involvement, what kind of palliative filter is one talking about?

8. What Kind of Filter Would You Want?

There seem to be two ways one could involve a palliative support team in the euthanasia procedure. One possibility would be a prior consultation, not about the euthanasia request itself but only about possible palliative alternatives, a consultation that takes place as soon as the physician hears or even suspects that his patient is about to make a euthanasia request. The other possibility would be that the palliative support team would take the role of the second physician or would join him and would thus, in a later phase of the procedure, be asked to assess the euthanasia request of the patient. The Palliative Care Federation clearly opted for the first possibility. It suggested that the attending physician, as soon as he is confronted with a euthanasia request, consults with the palliative support team of his institution or region (in Belgium such a team is available anywhere) concerning the concrete possibilities of palliative care. So the Federation clearly suggests a compulsory prior palliative consultation, not an assessment of the euthanasia request in a later phase of the procedure.

Six arguments were given in favour of this prior consultation, six arguments which again are only briefly presented here.

1. It is best to have this palliative filter at the beginning of the euthanasia procedure, because in a number of cases this filter will make the rest of the procedure redundant (because for instance physician and patient realise that there might be another solution).

2. When you want to have an informed decision then it is necessary to have the information first, before. Only *after* the information has been given cam an informed decision be made.

3. It is psychologically indefensible only after both physician and patient have taken the hard decision to go for euthanasia, to come up with possible palliative alternatives.

4. It is evident that alternatives that are given that late, after the actual decision has been made, are no real alternatives anymore. Also purely medically this often seems the case.

5. When palliative care services were to assess the euthanasia request, all this could lead to a confounding of euthanasia and palliative care by the general public, and this certainly would not be a good thing for the desired increase of the impact of palliative care.

6. A prior consultation that is supportive, medically but also ethically and psychologically, supportive and not judgemental, would probably enhance compliance and reporting, because physicians are

confident that they have not overlooked any alternative and therefore do not feel threatened.

There is a clear difference between the task of the Dutch SCEN physicians (supra) and the palliative consultation the FPZV is suggesting. What the SCEN physicians do is indeed assess the euthanasia request of the patient, taking the role of the second physician in the euthanasia procedure. What the FPZV is suggesting is a prior palliative consultation and, has been argued in the previous paragraphs certainly not an assessment of the euthanasia request in a later phase of the euthanasia procedure. The SCEN physicians are no palliative care specialists. The education they have received in palliative care is limited. Moreover SCEN physicians see the patients too late in the procedure, at a time where possible palliative alternatives just come too late to be a real alternative anymore. Though good arguments can be given to have a SCEN physician rather then just a colleague as the second physician in the euthanasia procedure and though it would be useful to have similar specially trained physicians in Belgium too, it would be a big mistake to think that they would be capable of fulfilling the kind of palliative filter role we would think would be necessary.[19]

This idea of a palliative filter, conceived as a prior palliative consultation, was not only supported by the palliative caregivers united in the Palliative Care Federation Flanders. In its euthanasia advice of 17 November 2001 the Belgian National Order of Physicians explicitly endorsed this proposal. That politicians from all major parties subscribed to the concerns of the FPZV and were positive about this idea of a prior palliative consultation became very clear when the Commission for Public Health of the House of Representatives in January 2002 in its advice on the Euthanasia Act unanimously endorsed the amendment proposed by the FPZV. That however the Commission for Justice of the House of Representatives later simply disregarded this unanimous advice can only be explained by the strong political pressure not to change a single letter of the bill on euthanasia, because changing anything would mean that the bill would have to be sent again to the Senate and that this was seen as too risky (imagine the government would fall and Christian democrats would return to

---

[19] See the detailed discussion in B. BROECKAERT, 'Goede zorg voor de dood. Palliatieve consultatie bij elk verzoek om euthanasie [Optimale care before dying. Palliative consult for every euthanasia request]' in *Medisch Contact* 55(2000), pp. 1597- 1600.

power). For the same reason very minor and very formal, though not unimportant amendments to the law, including those suggested by the Council of State, were simply disregarded. Better to have an imperfect Euthanasia Act, than no Euthanasia Act at all, several politicians belonging to the political majority argued.

9. After September 2002

The entry into force of the Euthanasia Act on 23 September 2002 only served to intensify the process of reflection about euthanasia and other forms of medically assisted death within the FPZV and its various subdivisions. It was clear that several months after this among a large number of caregivers, there existed still a great deal of uncertainty and many questions regarding euthanasia and the Euthanasia Act. As the umbrella organization promoting Flemish palliative care initiatives, it seemed appropriate for the FPZV to publish a new position paper, taking into account both the new legal situation and its practical consequences and the concerns it had raised earlier.[20] In what follows I present the seven points made in this paper, which taken together, give a very good idea of the position the FPZV takes, in the context of a country in which euthanasia has become a legal possibility (this should always be kept in mind), regarding the relationship between palliative care and euthanasia.

1. Palliative care and euthanasia are neither alternatives nor opposites. When a physician is willing to comply with a euthanasia request made by a patient who continues to suffer intolerably, despite the best possible care, there is no abrupt break between the palliative care the physician had been providing up to that point and the euthanasia he now is to perform. On the contrary, euthanasia in this case constitutes part of the palliative care which the physician and the team of caregivers provide to the patient and his/her loved ones.

2. Dialogue and respect are crucial in dealing with euthanasia and other forms of medically assisted death. The best chances of a dignified death are ensured through an honest and interactive attitude

---

[20] FEDERATION PALLIATIVE CARE FLANDERS, *Omgaan met euthanasie en andere vormen van medisch begeleid sterven* [Handling euthanasia and other ways of medically assisted dying], Wemmel, 6 September 2003.

toward the patient, characterized by openness and the highest degree of respect for the beliefs of the patient and those of the physician and the other caregivers. With issues such as these, caregivers are fully entitled to set their own ethical limits, though they are expected to do so in advance, in an honest and clear manner.

3. People do not request euthanasia out of some morbid death wish, or because they have always wanted so much to die, but rather because at a certain moment in the process of their illness, the suffering, and consequently their lives, become too much to bear. Various factors can play a decisive role in this, often in combination: fear of what is to come, respiratory difficulties, physical pain, loss of control over bodily functions, increasing weakness and dependence on others, etc. So a request for euthanasia always has something to do with an existing or expected decline in one's quality of life as a result of the patient's physical, psycho-social or spiritual suffering. It is therefore the responsibility of a caregiver who receives a euthanasia request to get through successive open and in-depth discussions a fair idea of the reasons behind the patient's desire to end his/her life:[21] what is it exactly that makes the patient's life no longer bearable?

4. Given the delicate, irreversible and far-reaching nature of euthanasia, it is of the utmost importance that euthanasia only be performed when it is a matter of suffering "that cannot be alleviated",[22] and a situation "for which there is no other reasonable solution".[23] This is why the caregiver and the patient must investigate whether a 'normal' medical treatment might not be able to alleviate the physical, psychosocial or spiritual suffering which lies at the origin of his/her request for euthanasia. For example, when a patient requests euthanasia because the physical pain is no longer tolerable, euthanasia may only be considered when it is obvious that even optimised pain therapy is no longer of any benefit. A request to end one's life, even if it is still vague, must always give rise to an evaluation and, if necessary, an adjustment of the care regime. What might be done to gear the care even more to the needs of the patient? Is it really impossible to alleviate the patient's suffering? Or have we simply reached the limits of our own abilities and is specialized advice therefore required?

---

[21] Belgian Euthanasia Act, article 3, §2, 2°.
[22] *Ibid.*, article 3, §1.
[23] *Ibid.*, article 3, §2, 1°.

5. Because it considers human beings in their totality, palliative care is interdisciplinary by definition. For this reason, a physician who receives a request for euthanasia can never act alone when caring for this patient or when making a decision about honouring the euthanasia request. Dealing with a euthanasia request in a responsible manner always involves an interdisciplinary approach, for on the one hand, there are many diverse and complex motives which can underlie a request to end one's life, and there are various caregivers who can offer their own ideas about the issues. For instance, nurses are often very close to their patients, both literally and figuratively, and thereby they are often in a good position to know what is lacking. It is clear, on the other hand, that specialized input from various disciplines is often necessary in order to alleviate the patient's suffering.

6. Due to the important role played by specialized and interdisciplinary expertise, it is strongly recommended that the local palliative team is consulted when a physician is confronted with an euthanasia request. In Flanders there exists a comprehensive network of palliative teams whose job is precisely to improve the frequently problematic quality of life of incurably ill patients, and to alleviate their suffering as much as possible, no matter what its nature may be. The interdisciplinary expertise and emancipatory approach used by these teams ensures their careful and efficient action. When a physician or caregiver receives a euthanasia request, these teams are ready and willing to provide palliative expertise, not to make decisions in their place but to inform them about the various palliative options and to offer them support. In this way, the tragedies associated with false choices, which have more to do with a lack of good palliative care than with an express wish to end one's life, can be prevented, thus making the choice of euthanasia a genuine informed choice. Consequently, the FPZV reiterates its suggestion to include within the euthanasia procedure a prior palliative consultation with the palliative team from one's own institution or from the local palliative network. Experience has shown by the way that many physicians, rightly concerned about making a responsible decision when confronted with a euthanasia request, do assign an important role to the consultation with the palliative team — just as they do in the case of other delicate ethical questions surrounding the end of life.

7. Caregivers can direct all their questions concerning the end of life to the palliative teams. They, and their patients, may expect palliative

teams not only to supply information about possible palliative alternatives and to provide palliative support where needed; caregivers and patients may also resort to palliative networks and teams for information and support with a direct and specific connection with euthanasia and the Euthanasia Act. Physicians on the team can take on the role of the other 'second opinion' physician in the euthanasia procedure. What may *not* be expected of organized palliative care, however, is that it would substitute for the attending physician and, if needed, perform euthanasia in his/her place. This would be an utter denial of the emphasis we wish to place on the continuity of care and the emancipatory concern which is entrenched in the very organization of Flemish palliative care: the fundamental principle that organized palliative care is there in order to provide information and support, not to act in place of regular care.

10. Palliative Sedation

When discussing the relationship between palliative care and euthanasia, we can, as far as the Belgian situation is concerned, not limit ourselves to a discussion of euthanasia and the Euthanasia Act alone. We cannot but spend a few paragraphs on palliative sedation, for during the hearings in the Belgian Senate at the time of the euthanasia debate (February-May 2000) various people spoke about sedation. While sedation was defended as a possible alternative to euthanasia, some senators thought that what was proposed was nothing but euthanasia in disguise. Later the Belgian Council of State in its advice on the Belgian euthanasia bill was asking critical questions too about sedation. In Belgium too sedation became a cause of controversy.

In order to avoid a number of pitfalls present in such terms as terminal sedation and controlled sedation, from 2000 onwards Broeckaert introduced the term 'palliative sedation'.[24] By now, 'palliative sedation' has become the new standard term in Belgium, and is also

---

[24] See B. BROECKAERT, 'Palliative Sedation Defined or Why and When Sedation Is Not Euthanasia' in *Journal of Pain and Symptom Management* 20/6(2000), S58 (X). For a more elaborate ethical and conceptual discussion of palliative sedation, see B. BROECKAERT & J.-M. NUÑEZ OLARTE, 'Sedation in Palliative Care. Facts and Concepts' in H. TEN HAVE & D. CLARK (eds.), *The Ethics of Palliative Care. European Perspectives*, Buckingham, Open University Press, 2002, pp. 166-180; B. BROECKAERT, 'Palliative Sedation. Ethical Aspects' in C. GASTMANS (ed.), *Between Technology and*

quite well known in Europe: the session on sedation at the second conference of the European Association of Palliative Care (Lyon 2002) was entitled 'Palliative Sedation: Presentation and Discussion of Research Working Groups', and the EAPC Research Network has itself made a clear choice in favour of the term 'palliative sedation' in the guidelines it is preparing.

Having an acceptable term is of course not enough; we also need a good definition of what palliative sedation is. As palliative sedation is about symptom control, it would be a good idea to start our discussion with a definition of pain and symptom control. What is typical of pain and symptom control is not just the subjective intention behind what is done, but also and even more importantly, the adequacy, the proportionality of what is objectively done. Therefore, we would define pain and symptom control as 'the intentional administration of analgesics and/or other drugs in dosages and combinations required to adequately relieve pain and/or other symptoms'.[25]

Table 1[26]

	Flanders 1998	The Netherlands 1990	The Netherlands 1995
All deaths with End of Life Decisions — Physician Assisted Death	22 135 (39,3%)	39,4%	42,6%
Active Termination of Life	2 501 (4,4%)	2,7%	3,4%
Euthanasia	640 (1,1%)	1,7%	2,4%
assisted suicide	65 (0,1%)	0,2%	0,3%
without request	1 796 (3,2%)	0,8%	0,7%
Pain control with life shortening effect	10 416 (18,5%)	18,8%	19,1%
Withholding or Withdrawing of life sustaining treatment	9 218 (16,4%)	17,9%	20,2%

Humanity: The Impact of New Technologies on Health Care Ethics, Leuven, Leuven University Press, 2002, pp. 239-255.

[25] See B. BROECKAERT, 'Medically Mediated Death: From Pain Control to Euthanasia' in *13th World Congress on Medical Law. Book of Proceedings 1*, Helsinki, 6-10 August 2000, p. 100.

[26] L. DELIENS *et al.*, 'End-of-life Decisions in Medical Practice in Flanders, Belgium: A Nationwide Survey' in *The Lancet* 356(2000), pp. 1806-1811; P.J. VAN DER MAAS *et al.*,

Focusing on this adequacy or proportionality, — a clear match between the drugs given and the drugs needed —, is absolutely essential to differentiate pain control from euthanasia. That all this is not about splitting hair can be easily shown from the Dutch and Flemish figures on end-of-life decisions (table 1). Knowing that pain relief, even when heavy medication is given in extreme doses, is remarkably safe,[27] it is puzzling to read that both in the Netherlands and in Flanders in no less than 18,5 percent of all deaths nationwide, physicians have shortened the life of the patient while alleviating pain and symptoms with opioids.[28] If one takes a closer look at these figures, one learns that in 3 percent (4 100 cases in 1995 in the Netherlands) or even 5 percent (2 966 cases in Flanders in 1998) of all deaths nationwide, this pain relief with life shortening effect was 'also intended to terminate life'. One can assume that in these last cases, physicians often will not mind not giving an adequate dose or rather that they often deliberately — in order to terminate the life of the patient — give a higher dose than needed to relieve the pain. Here the importance of a good definition of pain and symptom control immediately becomes clear, for a doctor who willingly and knowingly overdoses, intending to terminate life, thus not respecting this notion of adequacy or proportionality, is not providing pain relief at all, but, without a shadow of doubt, committing (in)voluntary euthanasia

A clear definition of palliative sedation is extremely important too, for it helps to avoid confusion, — confusion again with euthanasia. In line with our definition of pain and symptom control, we define palliative sedation as 'the intentional administration of sedative drugs in dosages and combinations required to reduce the consciousness of a terminal patient as much as necessary to adequately relieve one or more refractory symptoms'.[29]

'Euthanasia and other medical decisions concerning the end of life' in *The Lancet* 338(1991), pp. 669-74; P.J. VAN DER MAAS *et al.*, 'Euthanasia, physician-assisted suicide, and other medical practices involving the end of life in the Netherlands, 1990-1995' in *New England Journal of Medicine* 335(1996), pp. 1699-1705.

[27] M. BERCOVITCH, M. WALLER & A. ADUNKSY, 'High dose morphine use in the hospice setting: a database survey of patient characteristics and effect on life expectancy' in *Cancer* 86(1999), pp. 871-877.

[28] DELIENS *et al.*, 2000; VAN DER MAAS *et al.*, 1991; VAN DER MAAS *et al.*, 1996.

[29] B. BROECKAERT, 'Palliative sedation defined or why and when sedation is not euthanasia' in *Journal of Pain and Symptom Management* 20/6(2000), S58 (X).

This new definition has been developed in order to overcome the limitations of the previous ones and incorporates the following elements. First, there is this often neglected but crucial notion of adequacy or proportionality. Sedation is certainly not just a matter of subjective intention. If a subjective intention to relieve a refractory symptom does not translate itself in an adequate and proportional intervention — 'giving as much as needed' — this stated intention is not the real intention or it is, we would say, real but perverted by other competing intentions. Whoever is knowingly and willingly giving more than is needed to relieve the refractory symptom is not doing sedation anymore, but performing euthanasia when this overdose shortens the life of the patient. On the other hand, whoever is clearly giving more than is needed, not knowing very well what he is doing, is, when his overdose shortens the life of the patient, guilty of medical malpractice. In neither case we are dealing with (adequate) palliative sedation.

Although the available clinical studies of sedation in palliative care provide more information on the various refractory symptoms that can give rise to the decision to sedate, and give an idea of the average length of sedation, the medication used and the dosage, many essential questions nevertheless remain unanswered, for instance: the question of whether or not sedation is to be combined with the withholding of artificial hydration and nutrition; the question of the way in which the decision to initiate sedation is arrived at, and the role played in that decision by the patient, the family and the health care team; the question of the relationship between sedation and euthanasia and the real practice of sedation *outside* the prestigious international centres for palliative care. There is an urgent need for further empirical research and, taking the empirical findings as a starting point, further ethical research in order to arrive in a satisfactory manner at solutions that will provide medical and ethical streamlining for this practice.[30]

---

[30] A large-scale research project coordinated by B. Broeckaert and P. Schotsmans will attempt to find answers to these questions. (funded by the Research Foundation Flanders, 2002-2004; a parallel Dutch research project is carried out at the University Medical Center St Radboud Nijmegen). See P. CLAESSENS *et al.*, 'Sedation for refractory symptoms in palliative care: an empirical-ethical study' in *Abstracts of the 8th congress for the European Association of Palliative Care*, 2-5 April 2003, The Hague, the Netherlands, p. 124.

Conclusion

The euthanasia debate in the Netherlands is now in its fourth decade. In recent decades, jurisprudence and regulations from the 'Royal Netherlands Association of Medicine' (KNMG, 'Koninklijke Nederlandse Maatschappij ter Bevordering van de Geneeskunde') have articulated the requirements that have now been adopted in the recent Euthanasia Act. The enactment of the law itself, in April 2002, did not give rise to intense debate since it only sanctioned an existing practice that was already officially tolerated. But this does not mean that the debate is not under change. Starting with the opening of a small number of hospices and profiting from the input of many local, regional and national palliative care organisations, palliative care is now being put on the agenda. Some years ago, the debate on euthanasia could be described in terms of data and procedures. The Netherlands can thus be criticised for having walked back to front. The euthanasia debate started at the end of the 1960s but the first hospices originated only in the early 1990s. Indeed, many problems remain there to be solved. Many physicians who are confronted with terminally ill patients still do not have adequate knowledge and expertise. Regulations securing thorough and careful consultation by specialists in palliative care *before* life terminating acts are carried out have not yet been developed adequately. The viability of sedation at the end of life and the question whether it can serve as an alternative for euthanasia deserves better empirical knowledge and more thorough ethical reflection. But on the other hand more and more voices can be heard, indicating that the euthanasia debate is widening and that, increasingly, attention is given to alternative palliative measures that can relieve a patient's suffering at least to a tolerable degree. The recent developments in palliative care thus give rise to optimism for the future. But optimism is a bad advisor if important problems that require urgent solutions are not addressed.

Compared with the Dutch debate, the Belgian euthanasia debate was very short. In Belgium the Euthanasia Act is not the result of a process that had been going on for decades, not at all. Only after June 1999 was it really started, after the Christian democratic parties, who had been dominating the government for decades, had lost the general elections. Whereas in the Netherlands palliative care became prominent at a time in which the euthanasia debate had in fact already been settled, in Belgium the development of palliative care preceded the euthanasia debate and the euthanasia regulations resulting from it. As a result Belgian (especially Flemish) palliative care could play and did play a very active role in the Belgian euthanasia debate, not comparable at all with the role played by organised palliative care or the attention given to palliative care in the Dutch debate. As a result of this the Belgian euthanasia debate itself could function as a lever that facilitated the further development of palliative care. Without the euthanasia debate, the role played by palliative care and the attention given to palliative care in this debate the budget of palliative care would not have been doubled in 2001. Though the recognition of the role to be played by the nursing team is an important improvement to the Euthanasia Act, it remains a pity that the compulsory palliative consult has not been incorporated in the Euthanasia Act. Nevertheless the efforts of the FPZV and the way it has responded to the euthanasia bills and the Euthanasia Act, have resulted in a very broad awareness that one cannot discuss euthanasia without also discussing palliative care, without thus putting euthanasia in this wider perspective. I have the impression that in most euthanasia protocols that have been developed in hospitals and nursing homes so far, this general palliative care perspective is clearly present; that in a large majority of these protocols the local palliative care team is given a prominent role. The National Council of the Belgian Order of Physicians in its most recent advice on palliative care, euthanasia and end-of-life decisions (22 March 2003) reiterated its view that in the case of a request for euthanasia as a rule the consultation of an expert in palliative care is appropriate. In any case, when confronted with a euthanasia request, in practice a lot of physicians seem to assign an important role to a consultation with the local palliative care team.

What the 'Flemish Palliative Care Federation' has published and what has been published here is not a plea for (or against) euthanasia or a plea for (or against) legalising euthanasia. The only thing we wanted to do is to argue that in a situation where euthanasia is very likely about to be legalised or is regulated (and that is the situation, very different form the situation in the vast majority of other countries, the FPZV is in), such legalisation or regulation is in any case highly problematic when palliative care is not made widely available and a prior palliative filter is not included in the euthanasia procedure. The only intention behind our plea for the inclusion of this filter in the Euthanasia Act and in euthanasia practice is the intention to ensure that in case of an euthanasia request palliative possibilities are utilized or at least thoroughly discussed, so that euthanasia is only administered when the patient genuinely wants it and tragic pseudo-choices resulting from poor palliative care, otherwise a distinct possibility, are avoided. In the circumstances we were in (we were going to have an Euthanasia Act anyhow) and are in (we do have it now), we thought the approach taken, though it is certainly not the easiest and most comfortable one, was the best way to take our professional responsibility for the very vulnerable incurably ill seriously.

References

BERCOVITCH, M., M. WALLER & A. ADUNKSY, 'High dose morphine use in the hospice setting: a database survey of patient characteristics and effect on life expectancy' in *Cancer* 86(1999), pp. 871-877.

BROECKAERT, B., 'Le cure palliative in Belgio [Palliative care in Belgium]' in *Bioetica e Cultura* 8(1999), pp. 45-54.

BROECKAERT, B., 'Goede zorg voor de dood. Palliatieve consultatie bij elk verzoek om euthanasie [Optimale care before dying. Palliative consult for every euthanasia request]' in *Medisch Contact* 55/45(2000), pp. 1597- 1600.

BROECKAERT, B., 'Medically Mediated Death: From Pain Control to Euthanasia' in *13th World Congress on Medical Law. Book of Proceedings 1*, Helsinki, 6-10 August 2000, p. 100.

BROECKAERT, B., 'Palliative sedation defined or why and when sedation is not euthanasia' in *Journal of Pain and Symptom Management* 20/6(2000), S58 (X).

BROECKAERT, B., 'Belgium: Towards a legal recognition of euthanasia' in *European Journal of Health Law* 8(2001), pp. 95-107.

BROECKAERT, B., 'Palliative Sedation. Ethical Aspects' in C. GASTMANS (ed.), *Between Technology and Humanity: The Impact of New Technologies on Health Care Ethics*, Leuven, Leuven University Press, 2002, pp. 239-255.

BROECKAERT, B., W. DISTELMANS & A. MULLIE, *Nota aan de Voorzitters en Leden van de Commissie voor de Volksgezondheid en de Commissie voor de Justitie (Kamer van Volksvertegenwoordigers)* [Memorandum to the chairmen and members of the committees of public health and justice (Chamber of Representatives)], Wemmel, 7 January 2002.

BROECKAERT, B., W. DISTELMANS & A. MULLIE, *Palliatieve zorg in de euthanasiewet. Open brief aan de Leden van de Kamer van Volksvertegenwoordigers* [Palliative care in the euthanasia act. Open letter to the members of the Chamber of Representatives], Wemmel, 13 May 2002.

BROECKAERT, B. & J.M. NUÑEZ OLARTE, 'Sedation in Palliative Care. Facts and Concepts' in H. TEN HAVE & D. CLARKE, *The Ethics of Palliative Care. European Perspectives* ('Facing Death' Series), Buckingham, Open University Press, 2002, p. 166-180.

BROECKAERT, B. & P. SCHOTSMANS, 'Palliative Care in Belgium' in H. TEN HAVE & R. JANSSENS (eds.), *Palliative Care in Europe. Concepts and Policies*, Amsterdam, IOS Press — Ohmsha, 2001, pp. 31-42.

BRUNTINK, R., *Een goede plek om te sterven. Palliatieve zorg in Nederland. Een wegwijzer* [A good place to die. Palliative care in the Netherlands. A guide], Zutphen, Plataan, 2002.

CLAESSENS, P., R. JANSSENS, R. REUZEL, H. TEN HAVE, B. CRUL, P. SCHOTSMANS & B. BROECKAERT, 'Sedation for refractory symptoms in palliative care: an empirical-ethical study' in *Abstracts of the 8th congress of the European Association for Palliative Care*, 2-5 April 2003, The Hague, the Netherlands, p. 124.

DELIENS, L., F. MORTIER, J. BILSEN, M. COSYNS, R. VANDER STICHELE, J. VANOVERLOOP & K. INGELS, 'End-of-life Decisions in Medical Practice in Flanders, Belgium: A Nationwide Survey' in *The Lancet* 356(2000), pp. 1806-1811.

DEPARTMENT OF HEALTH, WELFARE AND SPORTS, *Palliatieve zorg in de terminale fase* [Palliative care in the terminal phase], Letter to the Chairman of the House of Representatives of the States General, 18 April 1996.

DEPARTMENT OF HEALTH, WELFARE AND SPORTS, *Definitief standpunt palliatieve zorg* [Final position on palliative care], Letter to the Chairman of the House of Representatives of the States General, 11 March 2002.

FEDERATION PALLIATIVE CARE FLANDERS, *Palliatieve zorg, euthanasie en menswaardig sterven. Standpuntbepaling naar aanleiding van de op 20 december ingediende wetsvoorstellen betreffende euthanasie en palliatieve zorg* [Palliative care, euthanasia and dying with dignity. Position statement in response to the bills on euthanasia and palliative care submitted on 20 December], Wemmel, 27 January 2000.

FEDERATION PALLIATIVE CARE FLANDERS, *Federatie Palliatieve Zorg Vlaanderen pleit voor een palliatieve filter in de euthanasieprocedure* [Federation palliative care Flanders pleads for a palliative filter in the euthanasia procedure], Wemmel, 26 September 2001.

FEDERATION PALLIATIVE CARE FLANDERS, *Omgaan met euthanasie en andere vormen van medisch begeleid sterven* [Handling euthanasia and other ways of medically assisted dying], Wemmel, 6 September 2003.

HOUSE OF REPRESENTATIVES OF THE STATES GENERAL, *Toetsing van levensbeëindiging op verzoek en hulp bij zelfdoding en wijziging van het Wetboek van Strafrecht en van de Wet op de Lijkbezorging (26 691)* [Review of life termination on request and assisted suicide and amendment of the criminal code and the burial and cremation act], Letter of the Minister of Health, Welfare and Sports, no. 44, 22 November 2001.

Janssens, R., *Palliative care. Concepts and ethics,* Nijmegen, Nijmegen University Press, 2001.

Janssens, R., P. Claessens, R. Reuzel, H. ten Have, B. Broeckaert, P. Schotsmans & B. Crul, 'The ethics of decision-making when suffering has become refractory. The case of Belgium and the Netherlands' in *Abstracts of the 8th congress of the European Association for Palliative Care*, 2-5 April 2003, The Hague, the Netherlands, p. 94.

Janssens, R., H. ten Have, D. Clark, B. Broeckaert, D. Gracia, F.J. Illhardt, G. Lantz, S. Privitera & P. Schotsmans, 'Palliative care in Europe. Towards a more comprehensive understanding' in *European Journal of Palliative Care* 8(2001), pp.20-23.

Janssens, R., H. ten Have & Z. Zylicz, 'Hospice and euthanasia in the Netherlands. An ethical point of view' in *Journal of Medical Ethics* 25(1999), pp. 408-412.

Janssens, R., A. Wijn, Z. Zylicz, H. Ten Have, R. Reuzel & B. Crul, 'Controversen rondom terminale sedatie [Controversies on terminal sedation]' in *Tijdschrift voor Geneeskunde en Ethiek* 12(2002), pp. 79-83.

Oostveen, M., 'Spijt. Voorvechters van de euthanasiepraktijk bezinnen zich [Remorse. Proponents of euthanasia reorient themselves]' in *NRC Handelsblad*, 10 November 2001.

ten Have, H. & R. Janssens, 'Toetsing van euthanasie. Verbetering terminale zorg noodzakelijk [Review of euthanasia. Optimisation of terminal care is necessary]' in *Christen Democratische Verkenningen* 5(1997), pp.186-193.

van der Maas, P.J., J.J.M. van Delden, L. Pijnenborg & C.W.N. Looman, 'Euthanasia and other medical decisions concerning the end of life' in *The Lancet* 338(1991), pp. 669-74;

van der Maas, P. J., G. van der Wal, I. Haverkate, C.L.M. de Graaff, J.G.C. Kester, B.D. Onwuteaka-Philipsen, A. van der Heide, J.M. Bosma & D.L. Willems, 'Euthanasia, physician-assisted suicide, and other medical practices involving the end of life in the Netherlands, 1990-1995' in *New England Journal of Medicine* 335(1996), pp. 1699-1705.

van der Wal, G. & P.J. van der Maas, *Euthanasie en andere medische beslissingen rond het levenseinde* [Euthanasia and other medical decisions at the end of life], Den Haag, Sdu, 1996.

Zylicz, Z., 'Hospice in Holland. The story behind the blank spot' in *American Journal of Hospice and Palliative Care* 4(1993), pp. 30-34.

REPORTING EUTHANASIA
PHYSICIANS' EXPERIENCES WITH A DUTCH REGIONAL EVALUATION COMMITTEE

Marta van Dijk, Guy A.M. Widdershoven
& Agnes M. Meershoek

Introduction

In the Netherlands, physicians who have carried out euthanasia or physician assisted suicide (PAS) are not prosecuted, provided that they have met the requirements of due care as laid down in the Euthanasia Act. According to these requirements, the physician has to be convinced that the patient's request to have his life ended is voluntary and well considered and that the patient suffers unbearably, without prospect of improvement. Next to this, the physician has to inform the patient about his conditions and prospects and he has to agree with the patient that there is no other reasonable way to relieve his suffering. Furthermore, the physician has to consult at least one other independent physician, who visits the patient and gives his opinion in writing on the patient's condition and his request to die. Finally, euthanasia or PAS has to be carried out medically careful, preferably in accordance with the guidelines the Royal Dutch Society for Pharmacology (KNMP) has formulated on this subject. In addition, physicians are requested by law to report a case of euthanasia or PAS.

A study conducted in the mid-1990s indicated that six out of ten physicians did not report euthanasia.[1] This was a matter of concern to the government, since a low report percentage interferes with controlling and improving the practice of euthanasia. Regional evaluation

---

[1] G. VAN DER WAL & P.J. VAN DER MAAS, *Euthanasie en andere medische beslissingen rond het levenseinde. De praktijk en de meldingsprocedure* [Euthanasia and other medical decisions concerning the end of life. The practice and the notification procedure], 's Gravenhage, Sdu, 1996.

committees on euthanasia were considered to be a solution to this problem. Five committees, composed of a legal specialist, a physician and an expert on ethical or philosophical issues, were established in 1998. They judge whether physicians who have carried out euthanasia or PAS have met the requirements of due care. The evaluation committees were expected to increase the willingness to report among physicians. Judgement of a physician's course of action is no longer a strictly juridical procedure, as physicians take part in the committees to represent the medical point of view. Furthermore, the committees can be regarded as a buffer between physicians and the public prosecutor. Because of this it was thought that physicians would have fewer qualms about reporting euthanasia. Nevertheless the number of reported cases has remained stable.[2] Considering the above-mentioned, it is interesting to explore physicians' experiences with the evaluation committees. In view of this, twelve physicians (general practitioners as well as medical specialists) were interviewed.[3] These physicians have reported a case of euthanasia to the evaluation committee in the region of Noord-Brabant and Limburg. Six physicians were selected and the evaluation committee requested them to give more information about their reports by telephone. Six other physicians, who were not asked to go into their reports in more detail, were also included in the study. Two of the interviewed general practitioners are so-called SCEN physicians. They have been trained to advise physicians who are confronted with a patient who requests euthanasia. The results of the study will be described following the order of the evaluation procedure as carried out by the evaluation committee. Finally, the results will be discussed.

1. Report Form

After having carried out euthanasia or PAS, a physician fills in a report form. This form contains questions about the patient's

---

[2] REGIONALE TOETSINGSCOMMISSIES EUTHANASIE, Jaarverslagen 1999, 2000, 2001 [Regional Evaluation Committees on Euthanasia, Annual Reports 1999, 2000, 2001], to be found at http://www.minvws.nl and http://www.minjus.nl.

[3] M. VAN DIJK, Ervaringen van artsen met de werkwijze van de regionale toetsingscomssisies euthanasie (regio Noord-Brabant en Limburg), [Physician's experiences with the procedure of the regional evaluation committees on euthanasia (region of Noord-Brabant and Limburg)], MA Thesis Health Sciences, University of Maastricht, 2002.

suffering, his request for euthanasia or PAS, the consultation of another physician and the way in which euthanasia or PAS has been carried out. By means of the report form physicians can also bring other important information to the attention of the evaluation committee. In general, physicians who took part in the study valued the report form positively. They said the questions that had to be answered link up well with the circumstances they face when a patient asks to have his life ended. However, some physicians thought it can be difficult for the evaluation committee to assess a physician's course of action only on the basis of a report form, without having contacted the patient. Not all physicians found it easy to make unequivocally clear why they have decided to comply with a request for euthanasia. Next to this, some physicians said that filling in the report form is time-consuming and roundabout. In their opinion, the information they provided in the report form largely overlaps with the patient's medical file, which is also sent to the committee.

2. Judging a Report

In addition to the report form and the patient's medical file, the evaluation committee receives the statement of the consulted physician and the patient's will concerning the end of his life. On the basis of this information the committee judges whether a physician has met the requirements of due care. Sometimes the committee is in doubt about this or needs more information in order to reach a decision. If so, the committee will ask the physician to amplify his report, either in writing or by telephone. In exceptional cases this still does not enable the evaluation committee to decide whether the requirements of due care have been met. The physician will then be invited to a committee meeting in order to clarify his course of action in person. In nearly all cases the evaluation committees conclude that the requirements of due care have been met. Only if these requirements have not been met will the report be forwarded to the public prosecutor.

Those physicians who had been asked to amplify on their report by telephone received a call by the physician of the evaluation committee. The physicians appreciated the open and understanding attitude of the committee's physician during these calls. Furthermore, they looked upon the physician as the obvious committee member to discuss their report with, considering the fact that the questions often concern the patient's medical condition. The physicians held different opinions about the committee's request to clarify their course of action by telephone. One of them deemed the request unnecessary. In his view, his report left no doubt whether he had met the requirements of due care. According to another physician the request to amplify on his report indicated that the evaluation committee proceeds very carefully in performing its task.

3. The Judgement of the Evaluation Committee

When a report has been received, the evaluation committee ascertains whether the requirements of due care have been met, usually within six weeks. The committee informs the physician with its judgement on his course of action by means of a judgement report. In this report, the patient's situation, his request to have his life ended, the consultation of another physician, and the way the physician has carried out euthanasia are also described. The interviewed physicians appreciated this report. Furthermore, they deemed the judgement to be formulated clearly.

Sometimes a physician's course of action can give the committee cause to make a comment, which is entered in the judgement report. Through this comment, the evaluation committee intends to change a physician's course of action the next time he receives a request for euthanasia. Two of the interviewed physicians got such a comment. One of them was not pleased with the comment. Taking the directions of the 'Royal Dutch Society for Pharmacology' (KNMP) into account, the evaluation committee concluded that the physician had administered an overdose of euthanatic drugs to the patient. The committee judged the physician's course of action as a whole to be careful, but commented that he had acted not entirely carefully with regard to the dose of euthanatic he had administered. The physician did not agree with this comment. To support his claim, he referred to the fact that he did act in accordance with specific directions, except these were other directions than those formulated by the KNMP. Apart from that, the KNMP directions are not binding upon physicians. In view of this the physician had asked the evaluation committee to withdraw the comment. The committee did not grant this request. This example shows that a comment will only be effective if the physician can go along with it.

Most physicians agreed with the composition of the evaluation committees. They all considered the physician as an indispensable committee member. Because of his medical experience, he was thought to be able to put himself in a physician's course of action as well as in the position of a patient. Some physicians said they had fewer qualms about reporting euthanasia, knowing their reports would be judged by a physician as well. Most physicians did not raise objections to a legal specialist and an expert on ethical or philosophical issues also taking part in the committee. They thought a legal specialist is needed because reviewing reports of euthanasia is a statutory procedure. Next to this, they said ethical considerations regarding euthanasia call for an expert on ethical or philosophical issues. However, a couple of physicians frowned upon a legal specialist and an expert on ethical or philosophical issues judging their reports. In their opinion, these committee members are not eligible to decide whether a physician has met the requirements of due care because they lack medical experience.

4. Requirements of Due Care

The requirements of due care were clear to all interviewed physicians. Nevertheless, physicians can find themselves faced with difficulties concerning the further interpretation of these requirements. For instance, it is known that a physician has to consult another physician when a patient requests euthanasia. The consulted physician has to visit the patient, but it is not always clear when exactly this visit should take place. For example, a patient who suffers unbearably is sometimes unable to speak due to his medical condition. If such is the case, a consulted physician will not be able to decide whether the patient's request for euthanasia is voluntary and well considered. Taking this into account, an interviewed physician asked the consulted physician to visit the patient when he was still able to talk about his condition and his request for euthanasia. Several months later, euthanasia was performed. In this case, the evaluation committee commented there had been too long a gap between the visit of the consulted physician and the moment euthanasia was carried out. The consulted physician should have visited the patient once again, shortly before the actual euthanasia.

5. Procedure of the Evaluation Committees

The interviewed physicians said the procedure that the evaluation committees follow when judging a report of euthanasia is clear to them in general. In particular the SCEN physicians were acquainted with this procedure. This is understandable: they had this information at first hand, as members of the evaluation committees play a part in the course physicians take to become a SCEN physician. Most other physicians said they had an overall picture of the procedure. Yet some elements appeared to be less well known. For instance, not all physicians knew the evaluation committee will not decide that a physician has not met the requirements of due care without having offered him the opportunity to amplify on his course of action in person.

Further information on the way in which the evaluation committees proceed when judging a physician's course of action can be found in their annual reports. These reports were mostly read by the SCEN physicians, who are already well informed on this subject. The other physicians hardly read these reports. Unfamiliarity with the procedure of the evaluation committees does not have to be an impediment to reporting euthanasia. Yet an interviewed SCEN physician said he knew from experience this unfamiliarity can be a reason why physicians fail to report.

6. Discussion

6.1. *Report form*

According to the interviewed physicians, the questions in the report form link up well with the circumstances they face when a patient requests euthanasia. However, physicians are sometimes confronted with situations which they either describe inaccurately or do not mention at all, since it is not always clear which information the evaluation committee exactly needs. Because of this, the report form does not always provide the evaluation committee with enough information to hold on to when judging a physician's course of action.

In view of the evaluation committee's decision process, it is important that a physician describes the patient's condition accurately. Yet the report should not be restricted to medical facts. It is advisable that a physician also focuses on the suffering of the patient. In addition, a physician should elaborate on the background of the request for euthanasia. In this way, the report supports a physician's decision to grant a patient's request for euthanasia. To the evaluation committee it can also serve as a kind of reference work which provides insight into a physician's course of action. As such, the report form facilitates the decision process of the evaluation committee.[4]

The report form contains a request to physicians to account for their answers. Next to this, it is said that physicians can add significantly to the committee's decision process by providing further information in the form of enclosures. However, it is questionable whether such terms sufficiently incite a physician to describe his course of action and the patient's situation in a way that would allow the evaluation committee to obtain a clear insight in the practice of euthanasia. This insight is very important to the evaluation committees, considering their objective to contribute to transparent and careful procedures in regard to euthanasia.

6.2. *Judging a report*

Physicians who were asked to amplify on their reports by telephone valued these calls positively. This can be ascribed to the attitude of the physician who spoke with these physicians on behalf of the evaluation committee. The views of physicians about the request to amplify on their reports by telephone correspond to results of a study conducted by Van der Wal et al.,[5] indicating that physicians either feel neutral about this request or value it positively. Not all physicians who had been asked to clarify their course of action by telephone saw the need for it, but they did not consider this request as a reprimand. They rather looked upon it as an opportunity to elaborate on their courses of action, so the evaluation committee could finally conclude they have actually met the requirements of due care.

---

[4] G.K. KIMSMA, 'Objectivering van de zorgvuldigheidseisen: mogelijkheden en problemen [Objectifying the requirements of due care: possibilities and problems]' in J. LEGEMAATE & R.J.M. DILLMANN (eds.), *Levensbeëindigend handelen door een arts: tussen norm en praktijk* [End-of-life acts by a physician: Between norm and practice], Houten, Bohn Stafleu Van Loghum, 1998.

[5] G. VAN DER WAL et al., *Medische besluitvorming aan het einde van het leven. De praktijk en de toetsingsprocedure euthanasie* [Medical decision making towards the end of life. The practice and the evaluation procedure], Utrecht, De Tijdstroom, 2003.

These views on the request to amplify on a report are in line with the committee's object of this request.[6]

To the public, asking a physician to amplify on his report by telephone may seem a rather obscure way to decide whether the requirements of due care have been observed. One might even question whether this course of action contravenes the public task of the evaluation committees. In view of this, it is important that the validity of the telephone call as a means to judge a physician's course of action is guaranteed. For that purpose, the telephone call does not have to be reshaped into a questioning, but it should be seen to that a physician's course of action is examined thoroughly. The call should be well structured. To ensure this, the evaluation committees have taken measures. For instance, prior to the telephone call a physician is informed in writing about the questions that will be asked. Furthermore, the physician who made the call on behalf of the committee draws up a report on it afterwards.[7]

6.3. *The judgement of the evaluation committee*

Most physicians appreciated it that the patient's situation and his request for euthanasia are described in the judgement report, as well as the consultation of another physician and the way the euthanasia was carried out. Physicians can conclude from these descriptions that the evaluation committee takes great care in examining their reports. They can also infer from the judgement report what information the committee exactly takes into account.

With regard to the judgement of the evaluation committee, it is remarkable that the course of action of a physician can be considered as careful, even though one of the requirements of due care has not fully been met. In an annual report of the evaluation committees a report is discussed concerning a physician who did not

---

[6] H. VAN DAM, 'Wij leggen een brug tussen praten over euthanasie en de praktijk. Gesprek met G. Widdershoven [We build a bridge between talking about euthanasia and the practice of euthanasia. Interview with G. Widdershoven]' in *Relevant* 26(2000)4, pp. 12-13.

[7] G.A.M. WIDDERSHOVEN, 'De werkwijze en de ervaringen van de toetsings-commissies [The procedure and the experiences of the evaluation committees]' in J. LEGEMAATE & R.J.M. DILLMANN (eds.), *Levensbeëindigend handelen door een arts op verzoek van de patiënt* [End-of-Life acts by a physician at the patient's request], Houten, Bohn Stafleu Van Loghum, 2003.

consult an independent physician. Instead he asked a physician whom he was associated with to visit the patient. The evaluation committee asked the physician to amplify on his report in writing. The physician stated that there was an important reason that made him decide to consult precisely this physician. His patient did not want to be visited by a physician she had never seen before. She only wanted to give a full account of her situation and her request for euthanasia to a physician she was familiar with. It so happened that the physician concerned was a near colleague of her general practitioner. On the basis of this amplification, the evaluation committee judged his course of action to be careful, in spite of the fact that he had not met the requirement of an independent consultation. The above-mentioned example illustrates that the evaluation committee takes into account that a physician sometimes cannot observe a specific requirement of due care when meeting a patient's individual needs.

Most physicians agreed with the composition of the evaluation committees. Only a few of them objected to a legal specialist and an expert on ethical or philosophical issues taking part in the committees. These views correspond with results of a study indicating that physicians generally approve of the composition of the evaluation committees.[8] Furthermore, it should be noticed that physicians, legal specialists and experts on ethical or philosophical issues look at a physician's course of action from a different angle. When a report of euthanasia is discussed, it is seen in a wider context due to the multidisciplinary composition of the evaluation committees. Because of this, a physician's course of action can be put in a new perspective. This adds positively to the decision process of the committees.[9]

6.4. *Requirements of due care*

The requirements of due care were clear to the physicians. Yet the further interpretation of these requirements sometimes caused difficulties. Considering the requirement of an independent consultation, it is

---

[8] J. KENNEDY, *Een weloverwogen dood. Euthanasie in Nederland* [A well considered death: Euthanasia in the Netherlands], Amsterdam, Bert Bakker, 2002.

[9] G.A.M. WIDDERSHOVEN, *Ethiek in de kliniek. Hedendaagse benaderingen in de gezondheidsethiek* [Clinical ethics. Contemporary approaches in health ethics], Amsterdam, Boom, 2000.

not always clear when exactly a consulted physician has to visit a patient. The chairperson of the evaluation committees acknowledges this can be a problem. She refers to a consulted physician who visited a patient at a moment the evaluation committee did not think the patient suffered unbearably. Two weeks later, the euthanasia was carried out. The chairperson wondered who regarded the patient's situation about this time, besides the physician.[10] This indicates that under certain circumstances a consulted physician should visit the patient twice, like an interviewed physician also found out. However, the requirements of due care are silent on this. Physicians find out about such a further interpretation of a requirement of due care in practice, for instance through a comment on this by the evaluation committee.

The way the requirements of due care have to be observed has not been laid down in detail. This adds to the discussion on this subject. In addition, it makes clear that these requirements cannot be met in a standard way. The way physicians can best meet the requirements of due care depends largely on their patients, whose conditions and individual needs differ widely.

6.5. *Procedure of the evaluation committees*

In particular the SCEN physicians were well informed on the exact procedure that the evaluation committees follow when judging a physician's course of action. Other physicians had an overall picture of this procedure, but some elements were less well known. After the evaluation committees were established, the willingness to report euthanasia among physicians was expected to rise considerably. Yet a substantial increase in the number of reported cases has failed to occur. Insecurity about what may happen when they report a case of euthanasia is one of the reasons why many physicians fail to do so.[11] The chairperson of the evaluation committees thinks the annual reports of the committees can acquaint physicians with the procedure, which subsequently will increase their trust in the evaluation

[10] H. VAN DAM, 'Vertrouwen winnen vraagt tijd. Gesprek met R. De Valk-Van Marwijk Kooy [Inspiring confidence takes time. Interview with R. de Valk-Van Marwijk Kooy], in *Relevant* 26(2000)3, pp. 6-7.

[11] G. VAN DER WAL et al., *Medische besluitvorming aan het einde van het leven. De praktijk en de toetsingsprocedures euthanasie* [Medical decision making towards the end of life. The practice and the evaluation procedure].

committees as well as their willingness to report.[12] However, these reports are mostly read by SCEN physicians, who are already well informed of the way the committees carry out the evaluation procedure. Other physicians hardly read the annual reports of the evaluation committees.

Information on the procedure of the evaluation committees can also be found in a government publication on the reporting procedure as regards euthanasia.[13] However, this information is not directed to what exactly physicians can expect from the evaluation committee after having reported a case of euthanasia. Therefore it might be advisable to distribute a leaflet to physicians in which the procedure of the evaluation committees is described concisely and clearly. Moreover, descriptions of reported cases and considerations of the evaluation committees when judging these reports could be published regularly in journals which physicians do read in large numbers.

The above-mentioned steps can contribute to the procedure of the evaluation committee becoming widely known among physicians, which may be conducive to their willingness to report euthanasia. A high number of reported cases is a prerequisite for the evaluation committees in order to contribute to transparent and careful procedures in the practice of euthanasia. This is a matter of major importance regarding the justification of the current practice of euthanasia on both a national and an international level.[14]

References

KENNEDY, J., *Een weloverwogen dood. Euthanasie in Nederland* [A well considered death. Euthanasia in the Netherlands], Amsterdam, Bert Bakker, 2002.

---

[12] H. VAN DAM, 'Vertrouwen winnen vraagt tijd. Gesprek met R. De Valk-Van Marwijk Kooy [Inspire confidence takes time. Interview with R. de Valk-Van Marwijk Kooy].

[13] MINISTERIE VAN VOLKSGEZONDHEID, WELZIJN EN SPORT & MINISTERIE VAN JUSTITIE, *De nieuwe meldingsprocedure euthanasie per 1 november 1998* [Ministry of Health, Welfare and Sports & Ministry of Justice, The new reporting procedure regarding euthanasia as of 1 November 1998].

[14] G.A.M. WIDDERSHOVEN, 'De werkwijze en de ervaringen van de toetsingscommissies [The procedure and the experiences of the evaluation committees].'

KIMSMA, G.K., 'Objectivering van de zorgvuldigheidseisen: mogelijkheden en problemen [Objectifying the requirements of due care: possibilities and problems]' in J. LEGEMAATE & R.J.M. DILLMANN (eds.),
Levensbeëindigend handelen door een arts: tussen norm en praktijk [End-
of-life acts by a physician: Between norm and practice], Houten,
Bohn Stafleu Van Loghum, 1998.

MINISTERIE VAN VOLKSGEZONDHEID, WELZIJN EN SPORT & MINISTERIE VAN
JUSTITIE, *De nieuwe meldingsprocedure euthanasie per 1 november 1998*
[Ministry of Health, Welfare and Sports & Ministry of Justice, The new
reporting procedure regarding euthanasia as of 1 November 1998].

REGIONALE TOETSINGSCOMMISSIES EUTHANASIE, *Jaarverslagen 1999, 2000, 2001*
[Regional evaluation committees on euthanasia, Annual reports
1999, 2000, 2001], to be found at *http://www.minvws.nl* and
http://www.minjus.nl.

VAN DAM, H., 'Vertrouwen winnen vraagt tijd. Gesprek met R. de
Valk–Van Marwijk Kooy [Inspiring confidence takes time. Interview
with R. de Valk–Van Marwijk Kooy]' in *Relevant* 26(2000)3, pp. 6-7.

VAN DAM, H., 'Wij leggen een brug tussen praten over euthanasie en de
praktijk. Gesprek met G. Widdershoven [We build a bridge between
talking about euthanasia and the practice of euthanasia. Interview
with G. Widdershoven]' in *Relevant* 26(2000)4, pp. 12-13.

VAN DIJK, M., *Ervaringen van artsen met de werkwijze van de regionale toetsingscommissies euthanasie (regio Noord-Brabant en Limburg)* [Physi-
cian's experiences with the procedure of the regional evaluation
committees on euthanasia (region of Noord-Brabant and Limburg)],
MA Thesis Health Sciences, University of Maastricht, 2002.

VAN DER WAL, G., A. VAN DER HEIDE, B.D. ONWUTEAKA-PHILIPSEN &
P.J. VAN DER MAAS, *Medische besluitvorming aan het einde van het leven.*
De praktijk en de toetsingsprocedure euthanasie [Medical decision making towards the end of life. The practice and the evaluation proce-
dure], Utrecht, De Tijdstroom, 2003.

VAN DER WAL, G. & P.J. VAN DER MAAS, *Euthanasie en andere medische*
beslissingen rond het levenseinde. De praktijk en de meldingsprocedure
[Euthanasia and other medical decisions concerning the end of life.
The practice and the notification procedure], 's Gravenhage, Sdu, 1996.

WIDDERSHOVEN, G.A.M., *Ethiek in de kliniek. Hedendaagse benaderingen in de*
gezondheidsethiek [Clinical ethics. Contemporary approaches in
health ethics], Amsterdam, Boom, 2000.

WIDDERSHOVEN, G.A.M., 'De werkwijze en de ervaringen van de toetsingscommissies [The procedure and the experiences of the evaluation committees]' in J. LEGEMAATE & R.J.M. DILLMANN (eds.), *Levens-*
beëindigend handelen door een arts op verzoek van de patiënt [End-of-life
acts by a physician at the patient's request], Houten, Bohn Stafleu
Van Loghum, 2003.

BEYOND AUTONOMY AND BENEFICENCE THE MORAL BASIS OF EUTHANASIA IN THE NETHERLANDS

Guy A.M. Widdershoven

Introduction

Euthanasia and physician-assisted suicide are controversial issues in medical ethics and medical law. In the debate, several arguments against the moral acceptability and legal feasibility of active involvement of physicians in bringing about a patient's death can be found. One argument refers back to the Ten Commandments: "Thou shalt not kill". Killing another human being is morally abject. According to the argument, this is certainly so for medical doctors, as can be seen in the Hippocratic Oath, which explicitly forbids abortion and euthanasia. A less apodictic argument refers to the slippery slope: if euthanasia would be permitted, a downhill movement is set in motion.[1] The end of this movement would be, on the one hand, that physicians will feel forced to assist people who ask for termination of life on whatever grounds. On the other hand, it might lead to a situation in which it becomes normal to kill people who are no longer useful for society.

In the literature and in the public debate, there are also arguments in favour of euthanasia and physician assisted suicide. One such argument invokes the right to die. According to this argument, decisions concerning life and death should be up to the individual concerned. In many countries, suicide is morally and legally accepted. If people are allowed to kill themselves, why should they be without rights when they are no longer able to perform the act themselves?

---

[1] J. KEOWN, *Euthanasia, Ethics and Public Policy: An Argument Against Legislation*, Cambridge, Cambridge University Press, 2002; H. HENDIN, *Seduced by Death: Doctors, Patients and the Dutch Cure*, New York — London, W.W. Norton & Company, 1997.

In medical ethics and medical law, patient autonomy is a central pivot. Patients have the right to refuse treatment even if this leads to their death. Shouldn't people also have the right to determine the moment of dying, if they are in a situation which is unbearable, and without prospect of improvement? Another argument focuses on the duty of the physician to alleviate pain and suffering. If there is no other option, the doctor, in fulfilling this duty, should be allowed to actively end the patient's life. This argument is not based on autonomy, but on beneficence.

The debate concerning euthanasia involves fundamentally different moral principles. This makes the debate interesting, if not central to medical ethics and medical law. Yet, the principles are normally presented in an abstract way. Discussants stick to very general ideas, which lack reference to specific social and historical conditions, and are not related to concrete experiences. To invoke the Ten Commandments, or argue for a right to die, implies the use of universal standards, which tend to be general and empty. From a philosophical perspective, this type of argumentation can be criticized. Following Aristotle, ethics should be based upon experience. Ethical knowledge requires participation in concrete practices. Central to ethics is a feeling for the concrete situation, which is always contingent and historical. From this perspective, it makes sense to consider how practitioners in specific situations deal with moral issues, for instance concerning euthanasia. What role do they give to notions such as autonomy and beneficence, how do they interpret them and apply them to the concrete situation?

In this paper I will present the Dutch experience with euthanasia. I will focus upon the way in which, during the past thirty years, the arguments in favour of euthanasia have been developed in interaction with euthanasia practice. I will show that patient autonomy has been a crucial pivot. Yet, the Dutch interpretation of autonomy is not purely liberal. It does not only involve rights, but also obligations. Next, I will make clear that the physician plays a central role, in that the moral and legal basis of euthanasia is a conflict of duties on the side of the physician. This brings in the issue of beneficence. Yet the Dutch interpretation of the duty to help is not simply paternalistic. In Dutch health care, the physician-patient relationship is based upon deliberation and mutual agreement. Therefore, my conclusion will be that the Dutch practice of euthanasia has a moral ground, which goes beyond the traditional opposition between autonomy and beneficence.

1. The Development of Dutch Euthanasia Practice

For the last 25 years, euthanasia has been a topic of debate in the Netherlands.[2] During this period, a practice of helping patients to die has been developed which is unique in the world. Since 1971, court cases have opened the way to euthanasia. Jurisprudence on cases of euthanasia and public debate have helped to bring about a social consensus on what counts as euthanasia ('active ending of a patient's life by a physician on the patient's request') and on the conditions which make euthanasia acceptable. In 1984 the Royal Dutch Medical Association (KNMG) formulated so-called due care criteria. In the 1990s, two surveys were performed to establish the number of cases of euthanasia and other decisions concerning the end of life.[3] The relative number of cases of euthanasia has risen between 1990 and 1995 (from 1,8 percent to 2,4 percent). The percentage of cases reported to the authorities has also increased (from 1,8 percent to 41 percent).

One of the major reasons for not reporting cases appears to be that physicians feel threatened by the procedure, outlined in the Law on Burial of 1994, in which the cases are evaluated by the public prosecutor. Very few cases are ultimately brought to court, but the procedure is unclear and time-consuming. It can also be doubted whether court decisions are the best way to develop a good practice of euthanasia. Therefore, a new policy concerning reporting has been developed. As a part of the new procedure, five regional multidisciplinary committees were installed in November 1998, which are to evaluate the cases that have been reported to the authorities.

Since April 2002, the law gives doctors who terminate life on request an exemption from liability if they have acted in line with due care criteria and have notified death by non-natural causes to the regional euthanasia review committee. According to the criteria, a doctor must be satisfied that the patient's request is voluntary and well considered, and that the patient's suffering is unbearable. Furthermore the doctor should inform the patient about the situation, discuss this and come to the joint conclusion that there is no other

---

[2] D.C. Thomasma et al. (eds.), *Asking to Die: Inside the Dutch Debate on Euthanasia*, Dordrecht — Boston — London, Kluwer, 1998.

[3] P.J. Van der Maas et al., 'Euthanasia and other medical decisions concerning the end of life' in *The Lancet* 338(1991), pp. 669-674; G. Van der Wal et al., 'Evaluation of the notification procedure for physician assisted death in the Netherlands' in *New England Journal of Medicine* 335(1996), pp. 1706-1711.

reasonable solution, consult at least one other independent physician who must see the patient and declare in writing that the aforementioned criteria are met, and exercise due medical care in the termination of life. Since the law on euthanasia has become valid, a positive judgement by a regional evaluation committee means that no further action is taken against the doctor.

2. Patient Autonomy in Dutch Euthanasia Practice

The background of the euthanasia debate and euthanasia practice in the Netherlands is the growing critique of paternalism in the second half of the twentieth century. A pivotal role was played by J.H. Van den Berg. In 1969 he published a small book under the title *Medische macht en medische ethiek* (Medical power and medical ethics).[4] He argued that as a result of the development of technology, medical doctors had become much more powerful. They were able to keep patients alive who would certainly have died in former times. This, according to Van den Berg, raised problems for medical ethics. Since Hippocrates, physicians were morally trained to make decisions in the interest of the patient. Patients themselves were supposed not to be able to take part in decision-making (because they are frail and vulnerable). Moreover, physicians should try to keep patients alive. The value of life is a central element in Hippocratic ethics; shortening or actively ending a patient's life is clearly immoral. As a result of the combination of new technology and old medical ethics, patients were being kept alive under inhumane conditions. Van den Berg argued in favour of a new medical ethics, which should acknowledge that quality of life is more important than quantity. This new ethics should give patients a say in crucial decisions, since they are more able than physicians to make judgements about quality of life. According to Van den Berg, active ending of life should no longer be a taboo in medical ethics.

In the years following the publication of Van den Berg's booklet, patient's rights became an issue in Dutch health care. In line with international developments, the right to refuse treatment was gradually acknowledged. More than in other western countries, the public

---

[4] J.H. VAN DEN BERG, *Medische macht en medische ethiek* [Medical power and medical ethics], Nijmegen, Callenbach, 1969.

and the medical profession came to share the idea that medical interventions should not be performed at all costs. In this situation, euthanasia became a relevant issue for debate. At first, the concept of euthanasia included all kinds of decisions concerning the end of life. No distinction was being made between active and passive euthanasia, or between decisions based upon a patient's request and decisions without it. In the 1970s, these distinctions were gradually introduced. H.J.J. Leenen, a central figure in the field of health law, played a crucial role. He argued that the concept of euthanasia should be used only in cases of active ending of life by a physician at the explicit request of the patient. Thus, euthanasia was distinguished from other medical decisions concerning the end of life, such as medical treatment with the shortening of life as a secondary effect, or active ending of life without a patient's request.

The Dutch debate on end-of-life decisions and the resulting definition of euthanasia as active ending of life at the patient's request made patient autonomy a central issue in the debate in more than one way. In the first place, euthanasia became linked to the notion of patient emancipation. In the second place, the patient's wish became a necessary condition. Thus, it may seem as though patient autonomy is the major moral basis for euthanasia in the Netherlands. Several participants in the Dutch debate on euthanasia have taken this position. The Dutch Society for Voluntary Euthanasia (NVVE) has regularly referred to the right to die as a justification for the legalization of euthanasia. The same organization has also emphasized that a person other than the patient cannot establish the condition of unbearable suffering. Whereas the physician should corroborate that the patient's suffering cannot be treated, and that the situation is without any prospect of improvement, only the patient can determine whether it can no longer be endured. Prominent ethicists in the euthanasia debate have supported this line of argumentation. It seems as though euthanasia in the Netherlands is the final outcome of the rise of patient autonomy and the upsurge of liberalism in medical ethics and medical practice.

Yet, this conclusion is too facile. In the first place, the Dutch have a specific view of patient autonomy. In Dutch health-care practice, patient autonomy is not primarily seen as the right to decide for oneself without any external interference. This notion of autonomy, which can also be described in terms of negative freedom[5], does play

---

[5] I. Berlin, *Four Essays on Liberty*, Oxford, Oxford University Press, 1969.

a role in health law in the Netherlands, which emphasizes protection of the patient against medical infringements. Yet, in medical practice a different notion of autonomy is to be found. The Dutch expect patients to act in a responsible way. In the euthanasia debate, the prevailing notion of autonomy is 'responsible autonomy'.[6] Thus, elements of positive freedom are crucial to the debate. The focus is not on freedom to make one's own decisions, but on deciding in a way which shows consideration for others. This is also apparent in the requirements of due care, which have been developed by the Royal Dutch Medical Association and have become codified in the Dutch law on euthanasia. In the law it is stated that the patient's request should be durable and well considered. Although it is not stated what kind of consideration is required, it is clear that patients are to take into account the consequences of their requests. The request should be discussed with the physician. In the context of Dutch health care, in which the physician performing euthanasia is supposed to know the patient (and in most cases acts as a family physician), such discussions are expected to involve more than just the affirmation that one really wishes the euthanasia to be performed. Concerning the issue of suffering, it may be doubted whether it is totally up to the patient to decide what counts as unbearable. Dutch physicians will not be satisfied with a simple declaration by the patient on the subject of suffering. They will interpret such declarations in the context of the patient's total situation. Again, the law puts much emphasis on the physician. It is the physician who has to be convinced that the patient's suffering is both without prospect and unendurable. If one reads the law carefully, and takes into account the context of Dutch health care, it is evident that the concept of patient autonomy plays a quite specific and also limited role in euthanasia in the Netherlands.

3. The Role of the Physician in Decisions concerning Euthanasia in the Netherlands

If patient autonomy in the sense of self-determination is not the most central value in Dutch euthanasia practice, one may wonder which

---

[6] J. KENNEDY, *Een weloverwogen dood. Euthanasie in Nederland*, Amsterdam, Bert Bakker, 2002.

other values are involved. A likely candidate is beneficence. Beneficence is a central value in medical ethics, to be clearly distinguished
from respect for autonomy.[7] If a physician acts on the principle of
beneficence, he or she takes a paternalistic stance. The emphasis is
on what the physician considers to be good for the patient. Not the
patient's, but the physician's view of the situation is crucial. If the
views of physician and patient conflict, the physician's perspective is
regarded as the more important one.

It can be argued that beneficence plays a central role in Dutch
euthanasia practice. As remarked above, the physician has to decide
for euthanasia. The physician has to be convinced that euthanasia is
the only alternative left. Dutch critics of euthanasia have commented
that this means that the patient has little say in the process.[8] Proponents of euthanasia do not draw this conclusion, but they do emphasize the physician's responsibility. The Royal Dutch Medical Association, from early in the debate, has stressed the physician's key role
as the central actor in euthanasia. Euthanasia is acceptable only if the
physician is convinced that suffering cannot be allowed to continue.
It has been argued that in deciding for euthanasia, the physician acts
out of compassion or mercy.[9] These arguments point in the direction
of beneficence as a central value.

Yet once again, this conclusion is too simple. Several aspects of
Dutch euthanasia practice are overlooked if one regards beneficence
as the key moral element. In the first place, a crucial issue in the
debate resulting in the legal acceptance of euthanasia is the exceptional character of active termination of life by the physician. Whereas
beneficence is a common value in medical practice, in euthanasia
there is more at stake. Euthanasia requires a conflict of duties on the
side of the physician. The principlist approach, which focuses on the
balancing of beneficence with other values, is not really applicable to
the situation of euthanasia. It does no justice to the tragic aspects of a
situation in which there is no option but to end a patient's life in order
to prevent further suffering. Secondly, it can be doubted whether the

---

[7] T.L. BEAUCHAMP & J.F. CHILDRESS, *Principles of Biomedical Ethics*, Oxford, Oxford
University Press, 2001.

[8] H.A.M.J. TEN HAVE & J.V.M. WELIE, 'Euthanasia: Normal medical practice?' in
Hastings Center Report 22(1992), pp. 34-38.

[9] R.J.M. DILLMANN, 'Euthanasie: de morele legitimatie van de arts' in J. LEGEMAATE
& R.J.M. DILLMANN (eds.), *Levensbeëindigend handelen door een arts: tussen norm en praktijk*, Houten, Bohn Stafleu Van Loghum, 1998, pp. 11-25.

physician is the one who decides what has to be done on the basis of his knowledge about the patient's condition. Whereas the argument for autonomy mistakenly regards the patient as the one who decides, and overlooks the role of the physician, the argument for beneficence tends to disregard the crucial contribution of people other than the physician who performs the euthanasia. In Dutch euthanasia practice, the patient's role is more than agreeing with the physician's decision and undergoing the consequences. The patient is a partner in the process of gradually reaching the decision that euthanasia is the only option left. The second physician, who acts as a consultant, plays a further significant role. The physician consulted has an important say in the matter. He or she must visit the patient and check whether the patient's situation is such that euthanasia is justified. This involves not just a physical examination, establishing the patient's disease, as is the case in the Belgian law. In the Netherlands, the consulted physician also has to establish the nature of the patient's request (is it voluntary and well considered?) and the character of the patient's suffering (is it unendurable?). Thus, the second physician has to verify that all the necessary conditions are fulfilled, and thereby plays a role which goes beyond mere professional advice based on knowledge of the disease. The situation around euthanasia involves more aspects than the concept of beneficence can account for.

4. Beyond Autonomy and Beneficence

If neither autonomy, in the sense of self-determination, nor beneficence, in the sense of the physician deciding in the interest of the patient, are suitable to serve as the moral basis for Dutch euthanasia practice, what other values can be relevant in this regard? Some such values have already been mentioned. The Dutch expect patients to be responsible. They tend to see the relationship between physician and patient as a partnership. This means that decisions in health care are seen as joint enterprises, in which physician and patient come to a shared conclusion. The physician-patient relationship, which is prevalent in Dutch health care in general, and in euthanasia in particular, is in line with the deliberative model.[10] In this model, patients'

---

[10] E.J. EMMANUEL & L.L. EMMANUEL, 'Four models of the physician-patient relationship' in *Journal of the American Medical Association* 267(1992), pp. 2221-2226.

values are regarded as important, but also in need of discussion; in the process of discussing values, the physician plays an active role. The patient is supposed to be able to learn to take a responsible stance, helped by the physician as a teacher or friend. The deliberative model is fundamentally different from an approach in which patient autonomy prevails (the informative model) or an approach in which the doctor is supposed to know best (the paternalist model). The emphasis is not on the point of view of one of the participants (either the patient or the physician), but on the development of a new, mutual perspective. The model embodies the principles of hermeneutic dialogue.[11] This aspect of mutuality is pervasive in Dutch health care. It is clearly expressed in one of the due care criteria, in which it is stated that the physician should discuss the situation with the patient and that the discussion should lead to the shared conclusion that no other options are available.

The Dutch expect help and support from their physician. Patients want to be sure that they can rely upon their physician in hard times. They hope that their physician will not let them die in a miserable way. A central value in this respect is trust. Concerning euthanasia, trust not only means that one can be sure that the physician will not misuse his or her power. It means first and foremost that one can be sure one will not be left alone in a hopeless situation. Concerning end-of-life issues, fear of abandonment is more pervasive in the Netherlands than fear of unwanted interventions by the physician. Patients express the need to be cared for, and not to be left alone to die. The values of support, trust and care are central to Dutch euthanasia practice. These values are hardly considered in the current debate in medical ethics, which focuses on autonomy and beneficence. They are elaborated by alternative approaches, such as the ethics of care.[12] The ethics of care might provide a better basis for understanding the moral issues involved in Dutch euthanasia practice than medical ethics, which tends to oscillate between arguments from autonomy and arguments from beneficence.

---

[11] G.A.M. WIDDERSHOVEN, 'The Physician-Patient Relationship: A Hermeneutic Perspective' in R.K. LIE et al. (eds.), *Healthy Thoughts. European Perspectives on Health Care Ethics*, Leuven — Paris — Sterling VA, Peeters Publishers, pp. 69-80.

[12] A. BAIER, 'Trust and antitrust' in *Ethics* 96(1989), pp. 231-260; J.C. TRONTO, *Moral Boundaries: A Political Argument for an Ethic of Care*, New York — London, Routledge, 1993.

Central values in Dutch euthanasia practice cannot be reduced to the principlist canon of autonomy and beneficence. Responsibility, deliberation and care introduce moral concerns that are neither strictly liberal, nor strictly paternalist. The central position of such values in Dutch health-care practice might also put into question one of the central arguments against allowing euthanasia: the slippery-slope argument. In so far as the slippery-slope argument is based upon the idea that physicians might not be able to resist a patient's wish to die, or, alternatively, that patients may become increasingly at the mercy of others who decide that it is better for them to die, these arguments use the same notions of autonomy and beneficence as the proponents of euthanasia do. If such notions are not adequate to describe Dutch euthanasia practice, the slippery-slope argument is not as easily applicable as it is often thought to be.

Conclusion

By focusing on responsibility, deliberation, and care as central elements in the moral justification of euthanasia, Dutch euthanasia practice highlights moral concerns which get little attention in the current debate on euthanasia. Dutch euthanasia practice does not support the view that patient autonomy is the most important argument for euthanasia, as long as autonomy is equated with the right to self-determination. The right to decide for oneself, without interference from others, is not the ultimate value in Dutch euthanasia practice. Likewise, Dutch euthanasia practice does not support the view that paternalism can serve as a moral ground for euthanasia. Although the physician plays an active role, this does not imply that the patient is merely subjected to what is regarded as being in the patient's interest. The Dutch experience not only can serve as a correction to arguments in favour of euthanasia, emphasizing either autonomy or beneficence. It can also raise some doubts about arguments against euthanasia, such as the slippery-slope argument.

References

BAIER, A., 'Trust and antitrust' in *Ethics* 96(1989), pp. 231-260.
BEAUCHAMP, T.L. & J.F. CHILDRESS, *Principles of biomedical ethics*, Oxford, Oxford University Press, 2001.

BERG, J.H. VAN DEN, *Medische macht en medische ethiek* [Medical power and medical ethics], Nijmegen, Callenbach, 1969.

BERLIN, I., *Four essays on liberty*, Oxford, Oxford University Press, 1969.

DILLMANN, R.J.M., 'Euthanasie: de morele legitimatie van de arts [Euthanasia: the physician's moral legitimation]' in J. LEGEMAATE & R.J.M. DILLMANN (eds.), *Levensbeeindigend handelen door een arts: tussen norm en praktijk* [End-of-life acts by a physician: Between norm and practice], Houten, Bohn Stafleu Van Loghum, 1988, pp. 11-25.

EMANUEL, E.J. & L.L. EMANUEL, 'Four models of the physician-patient relationship' in *Journal of the American Medical Association* 267(1992), pp. 2221-2226.

HENDIN, H., *Seduced by death: Doctors, Patients and the Dutch Cure*, New York — London, W.W. Norton & Company, 1997.

KENNEDY, J., *Een weloverwogen dood. Euthanasie in Nederland* [Well-considered death: Euthanasia in the Netherlands], Amsterdam, Bert Bakker, 2002.

KEOWN, J., *Euthanasia, Ethics and Public Policy: An Argument Against Legislation*, Cambridge, Cambridge University Press, 2002.

TEN HAVE, H.A.M.J. & J.V.M.WELIE, 'Euthanasia: normal medical practice?' in *Hastings Center Report* 22(1992), pp. 34-38.

THOMASMA, D.C., T. KIMBROUGH-KUSHNER, G.K. KIMSMA & C. CIESIELSKI-CARLUCCI (eds.), *Asking to die: Inside the Dutch debate about euthanasia*, Dordrecht — Boston — London, Kluwer, 1998.

TRONTO, J.C., *Moral boundaries: A Political Argument for an Ethic of Care*, New York — London, Routledge, 1993.

VAN DER MAAS, P.J., J.M. VAN DELDEN, L. PIJNENBORG & C.W.N LOOMAN, 'Euthanasia and other medical decisions concerning the end of life' in *The Lancet* 338(1991), pp. 669-74.

VAN DER WAL, G., P.J. VAN DER MAAS ET AL., 'Evaluation of the notification procedure for physician assisted death in the Netherlands' in *New England Journal of Medicine* 335(1996), pp. 1706-1711.

WIDDERSHOVEN, G.A.M., 'The Physician-Patient Relationship: A Hermeneutic Perspective' in R.K.LIE, P.T. SCHOTSMANS, B. HANSEN & T. MEULENBERGS, *Healthy Thoughts: European Perspectives on Health Care Ethics*, Leuven — Paris — Sterling VA, Peeters Publishers, 2002, pp. 69-80.

DEATH, DIGNITY, AND THE THEORY OF VALUE

Daniel P. Sulmasy

The word 'dignity' arises continuously in the debate over euthanasia and assisted suicide, both in Europe and in North America. Unlike the phrases 'autonomy' and 'slippery slope', 'dignity' is used by those on *both* sides of the question. For example, the organizations most prominently associated with the campaign that culminated in the recent legalization of euthanasia in Belgium are the *Association pour la Droit de Mourir dans la Dignité* and *Recht op Waardig Sterven*. Yet when Belgium passed its euthanasia law, that nation's Catholic bishops declared, "All this is opposed to the fundamental respect for human life that lies at the heart of a society based on human dignity".[1] Or, consider the fact that the legislation that legalized assisted suicide in the U.S. State of Oregon., was called the 'Death with Dignity Act'. Yet opponents of assisted suicide in the United States, such as the Family Research Council, have declared that, "(t)he idea of assisted suicide is a poison pill that kills the dignity of a precious human life".[2] Over and above differences in translation, the word 'dignity' cannot mean the same thing in all four of the preceding sentences. It cannot be the univocal basis of moral arguments both for and against euthanasia and assisted suicide. A better understanding of this word would therefore help to bring clarity and insight to the arguments about euthanasia and assisted suicide in Europe, North America, and throughout the world.

---

[1] P. AMES, 'Belgian bishops condemn Parliament approval of Euthanasia Bill' in *Associated Press Worldstream*, International News, 17 May 2002.

[2] B. KNICKERBOCKER, 'Latest showdown over assisted suicide' in *The Christian Science Monitor*, 15 November 2001, p. 3.

1. The Importance of Dignity

Dignity appears to be an important word in ethics. It occurs five times in the Universal Declaration of Human Rights of the United Nations.[3] The European Convention on Human Rights and Bio-medicine also uses it 5 times, even including the phrase "Dignity of the Human Being" in the full title of the report.[4] Liberal rights theo-rists in the U.S.A. such as Ronald Dworkin have noted the funda-mental moral significance of dignity, yet decried its lack of clear meaning. Dworkin writes,

> Anyone who professes to take rights seriously, and who praises our government for respecting them, (...) must accept at a minimum, one or both of two important ideas. The first is the vague but pow-erful idea of human dignity. This idea, associated with Kant but defended by philosophers of different schools, supposes that there are ways of treating a man that are inconsistent with recognizing him as a full member of the human community, and holds that such treatment is profoundly unjust. The second is the more familiar idea of political equality.[5]

Dignity, then, seems to be an important word in moral discourse. However, Dworkin's complaint remains true in the euthanasia debate. The word 'dignity' is vague, and it is used in different ways by different speakers. Therefore, either some conceptual clarification of the word must be accomplished, or it should be expunged from moral discourse about euthanasia or anything else.

2. Dignity and Value Theory

Elsewhere, in attempting to bring some clarity to the concept of dig-nity with respect to moral issues in the care of the dying, I have

---

[3] UNITED NATIONS, *Universal Declaration of Human Rights*, to be found at *http://www.un.org/Overview/rights.html*.

[4] COUNCIL OF EUROPE, *Convention for the Protection of Human Rights and Dignity of the Human Being with Regard to the Application of Biology and Medicine: Convention on Human Rights and Biomedicine*, ETS no. 164, to be found at *http://conventions.coe.int/Treaty/EN/CadreListeTraites.htm*.

[5] R. DWORKIN, *Taking Rights Seriously*, Cambridge, Harvard University Press, 1977, pp. 198-199.

drawn a distinction between attributed dignity and intrinsic dignity.[6] In this essay, I will further develop these thoughts by grounding this distinction between attributed and intrinsic dignity in a more general theory of value, further refining the distinction, and making fresh applications, showing the relevance of the concept of dignity to the morality of assisted suicide and euthanasia.

Every ethical theory, implicitly or explicitly, requires a theory of value (*i.e.*, an axiology). Classically, values have been divided into two main types, instrumental values and intrinsic values.[7] An instrumental value is always a function of usefulness. X has instrumental value to the extent that it can be used to achieve some valued outcome. Intrinsic value is not a function of a thing's usefulness. X has intrinsic value when it is valuable in itself. Kant, in the second formulation of the categorical imperative, seems to place great moral emphasis on this instrumental/intrinsic difference, in a way that is importantly related to his own conception of dignity. "Act in such a way that you treat humanity, whether in your own person or in the person of another, always at the same time as an end and never simply as a means".[8] Nonetheless, I want to argue that the story of value, dignity, and ethics is really much more complicated than the instrumental/intrinsic distinction.

3. Intrinsic Value

The field of environmental ethics has required a deep and careful exploration of the concept of intrinsic value. Labouring to understand whether species have value independent of human beings, writers such as Holmes Rolston have helped to clarify that there are things that have value in themselves — value that need not be conferred by a valuer. This is the value that things have by virtue of their

---

[6] D.P. SULMASY, 'Death and human dignity' in *Linacre Quarterly* 61(1994), pp. 27-36; D.P. SULMASY, 'Death with dignity: What does it mean?' in *Josephinum Journal of Theology* 4(1997), pp. 13-23; D.P. SULMASY, 'Healing the Dying: Spiritual Issues in the Care of the Dying' in J. KISSEL & D.C. THOMASMA (eds.), *The Health Professional as Friend and Healer*, Washington DC, Georgetown University Press, 2000, pp. 188-197.

[7] N.M. LEMOS, 'Value' in R. AUDI (ed.), *The Cambridge Dictionary of Philosophy*, New York, Cambridge University Press, 1995, pp. 829-830.

[8] I. KANT, *Groundwork for the Metaphysics of Morals*, Ak 429, (transl. J.W. ELLINGTON), Indianapolis, Hackett, 1981, p. 36.

nature and place in the universe, a value that is independent of any human evaluation. Truly intrinsic values, according to Rolston, "are objectively there — discovered, not generated by the valuer".[9] Intrinsic value, in this sense, is the value that something has solely in virtue of its intrinsic nature. At least one kind of thing in the universe (*i.e.*, the human natural kind) is capable of making judgements of value. This entails a duty to recognize and respect the value of those objects that have intrinsic value. But no matter whether this value is recognized by external valuers; no matter whether there even *are* any external valuers, things with intrinsic value have value. The source of this value is in them.

4. Attributed Value: Instrumental and Non-instrumental

Values that require a valuer, I call attributed values. These values exist by virtue of the attribution of some being capable of attributing value to an individual object, natural kind, state of affairs, concept, or some other sort of thing. This is the value something has in relation to me, or to my group, or to my kind. As I noted above, the classical approach has been to distinguish intrinsic value from instrumental value. But this may be far too simplistic a classification. I want to argue that the primary distinction in values is between intrinsic values and attributed values. Instrumental values are clearly attributed values. However, not all attributed values are instrumental. For example, an automobile has instrumental value in the sense that it can help me to go where I value going. I attribute the instrumental value to the machine. However, I may still attribute sentimental value to a 1963 Mustang that no longer runs and therefore has no instrumental value to me or anyone else as a driving machine. The mere fact that the value of a 1963 Mustang is not instrumental does not entail that its value is intrinsic. The non-instrumental value of a Mustang is not objectively there to be discovered. This value is attributed by a valuer, even though it is not instrumental. It therefore seems that there are both instrumental and non-instrumental attributed values.

---

[9] H. ROLSTON III, *Environmental Ethics*, Philadelphia, Temple University Press, 1988, p. 116.

All attributed values admit of degrees. Some things will have more value in relation to the valuer than do others. Value may be attributed to a thing one day and not attributed to that same thing the next day, depending upon the context and the condition of the thing. For example, a snow shovel has value to me when it snows, but does not have the same value to me if I move to the Riviera. The attributed value of a thing can vary from valuer to valuer, or from one group of valuers to another (e.g. a culture, a nation, or the nature of the valuing entity).

5. Intrinsic Value and Natural Kinds

Intrinsic value would appear to pertain only to natural kinds, not to individual objects, classes of individual objects, or artifacts.

Artifacts have only attributed value. They are, by definition, made by agents who attribute value to them, and are sometimes exchanged between agents who also attribute value to them. Generally, this attributed value is instrumental. For example, a knife is made in order to serve the goals of its user by cutting other objects and bringing about some valued state of affairs. But an artifact may also have attributed non-instrumental value. For example, an antique knife may have sentimental value. Or a knife may have aesthetic value because of the beauty of its handle or the shape of its blade. These values require a valuer to attribute them to the knife, but they are not instrumental values in that they are not good only to the extent that they help to bring about valued states of affairs.

Intrinsic value is said to be the value that something has solely in virtue of its intrinsic nature. That is to say, intrinsic value is the value that something has in virtue of its being the kind of thing that it is. This means that the very concept of intrinsic value commits one to the concept of natural kinds.[10] If one were to propose that intrinsic value pertained to individuals rather than natural kinds, then the phrases "in virtue of its intrinsic nature" or "in virtue of being the kind of thing that it is" would be literally senseless, and the concept of intrinsic value would only be confused. If one were unwilling to

---

[10] For a good contemporary approach to the concept of natural kinds, see D. WIGGINS, *Sameness and Substance*, Cambridge, Harvard University Press, 1980, pp. 77-101. Natural kinds are characterized by law-like principles that collect together the actual extension of that kind around an arbitrary good example of the kind.

accept the concept of natural kinds, there would only be individually existing things of which properties could be predicated. Things could not then be 'the kinds of things that they are,' but only individuals that do or do not have certain properties. If the universe really were to consist only of individuals without natural kinds, then the only thing that could truly define each individual thing "being the kind of thing that it is" would be its bare existence. But if that were the case, then everything that exists would have intrinsic value in equal amounts, and one could not say that one thing had intrinsic value and another thing did not. This would render the concept of intrinsic value meaningless.

Truly intrinsic value could not pertain only to classes of individuals that share particular predicates. Intrinsic value, by definition, is the value that pertains to a thing by virtue of its being the kind of thing that it is. Classes of things, based solely upon predicable properties, cannot constitute an intrinsic nature. To see why this is so, consider the example of a diamond. Diamonds are valued as a natural kind because of the characteristics that are typical of diamonds as a natural kind — their hardness, brilliance, refractive capacities, etc. Certainly much of the value of a diamond is attributed — it is conferred upon these gems by human valuers. But part of the value of a diamond is intrinsic. It depends upon an individual diamond's being the kind of thing that it is. Suppose that someone were able to manufacture a fake diamond that had all of the characteristics of a real diamond that are deemed worthy of admiration. Suppose further that it were manufactured in such a way as to imitate a diamond so well that even the expert appraisers at the diamond market in Amsterdam were fooled. Suppose it were later discovered that the this gem were a 'fake'. It would still be in the class of those individual things that share all the valued predicates that are typical of genuine diamonds as a natural kind, but that would not be enough to give it the equivalent *intrinsic* value of a diamond. It would not be the kind of thing that a diamond is. In fact, a defective gem that belonged genuinely to the natural kind of diamonds would be more valuable that a "perfect fake."

The foregoing is not a proof that there are such things as natural kinds. I leave that to the cogent arguments of recent philosophers doing work in metaphysics.[11] However, it is an argument that if there

---

[11] See, for example, D. WIGGINS, *Sameness and Substance*; B. BRODY, *Identity and Essence*, Princeton, Princeton University Press, 1980, pp. 130-133.

is such a thing as intrinsic value, then it pertains to natural kinds, and if one is committed to the concept of intrinsic value, one must be committed to the concept of natural kinds.

One should note further that the intrinsic value of any individual member of particular natural kind is always equal to that of any other member of the same natural kind. Unlike attributed value, the intrinsic value of a thing does not admit of degrees, once one knows what kind of a thing it is. The intrinsic value of a thing does not depend upon its value to a valuer, or how it is perceived by a valuer, or upon any group of valuers. The intrinsic value of a thing would appear to be inalienable. Intrinsic value cannot be divorced from the thing itself.

6. Dignity and Intrinsic Value

While all members of a particular natural kind have equal intrinsic value, the intrinsic value of different natural kinds does appear to vary and admit of degrees. The intrinsic value of a grain of dirt and the intrinsic value of a human being would appear to differ. I want to argue that intrinsic 'Dignity' (with a capital D) is the word we use to refer to the highest level of intrinsic value that a natural kind can have. Just as there are two types of attributed value (instrumental and non-instrumental), so there are two types of intrinsic value (simple intrinsic value and Dignity). Dignity, in this sense of the word, belongs to those natural kinds that have certain typical characteristics that give them a particularly high intrinsic value. The kinds of dispositional predicates[12] that characterize natural kinds that have intrinsic Dignity include the highly developed species-typical capacities for language, rationality, love, free will, moral agency, creativity, aesthetic sensibility, etc. that characterize the human natural kind. This is of course not to say that there might not be other natural kinds that also have such highly developed species-typical dispositional predicates. On the supposition that angels were to exist, they would certainly have intrinsic Dignity. It is quite conceivable that somewhere out there in the unimaginable immensity of the universe

---

[12] For a discussion of the concept of dispositional predicates in relationship to natural kinds and ethical theory, see A.J. LISSKA, *Aquinas' Theory of Natural Law: An Analytic Reconstruction*, Oxford, Clarendon Press, 1996, pp. 96-100.

there might be natural kinds on other planets that have such highly developed species-typical capacities that one would say that they also have intrinsic Dignity. All creatures on the planet Earth have some sort of intrinsic value. In my estimation, however, none of these other natural kinds have such highly developed species-typical capacities for language, rationality, love, free will, moral agency, creativity, aesthetic sensibility, etc. that I am willing to say that their intrinsic value is actually Dignity. Certain sea mammals come close, and this might merit serious discussion. But it is important to note that Dignity is a threshold concept, pertaining to natural kinds, not individuals. Only natural kinds have intrinsic value. And only the judgement that a particular natural kind is characterized by the law-like generalizations that constitute this threshold enables one to say that that natural kind has intrinsic Dignity.

Presuming then that the only natural kind we know that has intrinsic Dignity is the human natural kind, one can then see that this is a further explication of what I have previously called "intrinsic human dignity".[13] Further, one can see that this is roughly the way the word 'dignity' was used by Kant when he declared that "humanity itself is a dignity"[14] and insisted that human beings be treated as ends in themselves and never purely instrumentally. Finally, it seems that this is the way the word 'dignity' is used in the Universal Declaration on Human Rights and in the European Community's Convention on Human Rights and Biomedicine. This intrinsic Dignity is the kind of dignity that one has simply because one is a member of the human natural kind — a member of the human family.

7. Non-instrumental Attributed Value: the Attributed Dignities

Confusingly, the word 'dignity' is also used to refer to attributed values. There is a very common cluster of such uses of the word 'dignity'. One says, for instance, that some action is undignified, or that some state of affairs has resulted in a diminution of one's

---

[13] D.P. SULMASY, 'Death and human dignity'; D.P. SULMASY, 'Death with dignity: What does it mean?' and D.P. SULMASY, 'Healing the Dying: Spiritual Issues in the Care of the Dying', note 6.

[14] I. KANT, 'The Metaphysics of Morals, Part II: The Metaphysical Principles of Virtue', Ak 462, in *Ethical Philosophy*, (transl. J.W. ELLINGTON), Indianapolis, Hackett, 1983, p. 127.

dignity. All of these uses refer to a non-instrumental value, yet these speakers are not referring to truly intrinsic value (Dignity with a capital D). They are referring to attributed, non-instrumental values. I will use 'attributed dignities' (in the plural with a small d) to refer to these attributions of non-intrinsic, non-instrumental value.

It is important to note that not all non-instrumental attributed values can be called 'attributed dignities' (see table). Ordinary discourse further restricts the way this word is used, making it a subset of the non-instrumental attributed values. First, the word 'dignity' is generally not used in attributing non-instrumental value to artifacts, but only to natural kinds. Second, the word 'dignity' is generally used in this attributive sense only with reference to natural kinds that have intrinsic Dignity in the first place. Bricks, for example, can have both instrumental and non-instrumental attributed value, but as artifacts they have no intrinsic Dignity. Thus, they can have no attributed dignities. Bricks have instrumental attributed value for their use in construction. But they can also have attributed non-instrumental value — aesthetic value for instance. One might appreciate the look of a brick façade. Or the surface of the bricks may be impressed with a particular design that is thought to be beautiful. These are non-instrumental attributed values. Yet bricks are not described as having 'dignity'. One might occasionally hear someone say that a house has 'dignity', but this is generally an indirect attribution of non-instrumental value to the builder or to the interior designer or to the owner.

Table 1: Classification of Kinds of Value

Attributed		Intrinsic	
Instrumental values	Non-instrumental attributed values	Simple intrinsic values-	Intrinsic dignity
	Attributed dignities		

Thus, discourse about 'dignity' in the sense of the attributed dignities (with a small d) appears reserved for natural kinds that have Dignity in the intrinsic sense (with a capital D). In general, then, since we are most secure in the judgement that intrinsic Dignity belongs to human beings, the word 'dignity' is reserved for discourse about human beings even in the attributed sense. These attributed dignities are thus a subset of non-instrumental attributed values, reserved for beings that have intrinsic Dignity (*viz.*, human beings). In this attributed sense, one speaks, for example, of visiting 'dignitaries'. One claims that a certain task is 'beneath one's dignity'. One speaks of a person 'behaving in an undignified manner'. All of these, and other non-intrinsic, non-instrumental uses of the word 'dignity', require a valuer — oneself or another person — to attribute the value. These uses of the word 'dignity' do not refer to the value that a human being has by virtue of being a human being. That is to say, they are not referring to intrinsic values. But neither are these typically instrumental values. They do not refer to the usefulness of a human being to oneself or to another. These attributed dignities contribute in important ways to human flourishing. A complete moral theory would relate these values to virtues in the context of a fuller account of human excellence. Attributed human dignities also refer to more than the preferences of individual human beings. But a discussion of these issues would take us far beyond the more narrowly confined discussion of dignity that is the subject of this essay.

So, as shown in the table, I will consistently use the phrase 'intrinsic Dignity' to refer to the special type of intrinsic value that belongs to those natural kinds that have the capacities for language, rationality, love, free will, moral agency, creativity, aesthetic sensibility, etc. that merit this designation. I will use the phase 'attributed dignities' to refer to the non-instrumental values that are attributed to members of any natural kind that has intrinsic Dignity.

8. Dignity and Ethics

The value of a member of a natural kind that has intrinsic Dignity entails significant moral meaning. The notion of intrinsic Dignity entails both self-regarding and other-regarding moral duties for beings that have intrinsic Dignity. One of the primary features distinguishing the intrinsic value of a natural kind that has intrinsic Dignity from other natural kinds that have only simple intrinsic value is a species-typical capacity for moral agency. All members of a natural kind that has intrinsic Dignity and are individually capable of exercising the moral agency that is a distinctive of their natural kind have moral obligations to themselves, to any other entities that have intrinsic Dignity, and to the rest of what exists. The following list describes some of these duties. This list is not meant to exhaust the fundamental principles of ethics. It is limited to those fundamental principles that are most directly connected to the theme of dignity. But these duties should be taken as sufficiently fundamental and general to be considered true principles. All members of a natural kind that has intrinsic Dignity and are, as individual members of that natural kind, capable of exercising the moral agency that in part constitutes the intrinsic Dignity of their natural kind, have the following duties:

P-I) a duty of perfect obligation to respect all members of natural kinds that have intrinsic Dignity.

P-II) a duty of perfect obligation to respect the capacities that confer intrinsic Dignity upon a natural kind, in themselves and in others.

P-III) a duty to comport themselves in a manner that is consistent with their own intrinsic Dignity.

P-IV) a duty to build up, to the extent possible, the attributed dignities of members of natural kinds that have intrinsic Dignity.

P-V) a duty to be respectful of the intrinsic value of all other natural kinds.

P-VI) a duty of perfect obligation, in carrying out PP-I-V, never to act in such a way as directly to undermine the intrinsic Dignity that gives the other duties their binding force.

While the language of these principles might seem unfamiliar to bioethicists, the concepts are quite familiar. The second formulation of Kant's categorical imperative might be considered a corollary of P-I. Together, P-I, P-II, P-III, and P-VI are often labeled Respect for Persons; P-IV and P-VI are related to Beneficence and Non-Maleficence; P-V is sometimes called Stewardship. Justice arises from the need to balance the requirements of PP-II-V.

It is also important to note that the duty to build up the attributed dignities of any human being is logically dependent upon the intrinsic Dignity of human beings. The *primary* duty is to recognize and respect that intrinsic Dignity. The duty of building up the attributed dignities of human beings is a way of concretizing the fundamental duty of respect for intrinsic Dignity. As David Velleman has argued, from an ethical point of view, there must be something more fundamental to ethics than interests, namely a reason to respect a fellow human being's interests in the first place. The question can be asked,

for example, why should I care that this person has lost independence that I have the capacity to restore? Velleman's answer is that
we seek to protect and promote a fellow human being's interests
because we first respect the human being whose interests they are.[15]
This fundamental respect is for intrinsic Dignity — the 'interest-
independent' value of a human being. Without this primary respect,
there is no basis for interpersonal morality.

9. Death, Illness, Health Care, and Dignity

It is certainly true that illness, injury, and death attack the attributed
dignities of human beings. A wide spectrum of these attributed dignities can come under siege. Lennart Nordenfelt has helped me to
see how truly plural are the attributed dignities at issue in chronic illness.[16] Those who are ill are often robbed of their station in life. They
can become less productive and even unproductive. They are often
forced to become dependent upon others. They must suffer the indignities of assistance with activities of daily living such as walking,
bathing, dressing, using the toilet, and eating. Their appearance can
change, and they can become less attractive. They may lose consciousness, even permanently. They lose control of their situations
and planning becomes very restricted. Illness and dying bring these
attributed indignities upon human beings.

The beneficent task of medicine, nursing, and the other health-care
professions is first and foremost to eliminate or forestall or prevent
or ameliorate the occasions of such attributed indignities that arise in
and through the alterations in corporeal function known as pathology and pathophysiology. But it should be obvious that this cannot
be a duty of perfect obligation. Death is inevitable and the medical
professions imperfect. Nothing is more certain philosophically. So, in
caring for the dying, some attributed indignities will be inevitable
and ineradicable.

The foregoing now allows us to understand how it is that the word
'dignity' has been used to argue both for and against assisted suicide
and euthanasia. Those who argue for 'death with dignity' through

---

[15] J.D. VELLEMAN, 'A right to self-termination?' in *Ethics* 109(1999), pp. 605-628.
[16] L. NORDENFELT, 'Dignity and the Elderly.' Abstract presented at XVIth European
Conference on Philosophy of Medicine and Health Care, Malta, 23 August 2002.

euthanasia and assisted suicide would appear to charge the health professions with the elimination of the attributed indignities that patients suffer, even if this requires the elimination of the one who is suffering them. In so doing, according to the schema I have outlined above, proponents of euthanasia and assisted suicide who base their arguments upon 'dignity' are using the word in the attributed sense.

Those who invoke the word 'dignity' to argue against euthanasia and assisted suicide appear to use the word in the sense of intrinsic Dignity. They are not unaware of the ways in which illness, injury, and death affect the attributed dignities of human beings. Neither they nor their opponents dispute that the healing professions have beneficent duties with respect to the occasions of attributed indignities. No one on either side of the debate is against the role of palliative care, hospice, and other modalities of treatment that help patients to maintain their appearance and independence and maximize the possibilities for quality of life even while dying. However, opponents of euthanasia and physician-assisted suicide invoke the sixth of the moral principles noted above (P-VI) and argue that there are moral limits to the beneficent duties of health-care professionals. One of these limits is that one should never, in attempting to build up the attributed dignities of a person, act in such a way as to undermine the intrinsic Dignity that is the basis for these attributed dignities in the first place. They hold that euthanasia and assisted suicide do exactly this, and therefore cannot be allowed.

10. The Argument Against Euthanasia on the Basis of Intrinsic Dignity

The logical structure of the argument against euthanasia and physician-assisted suicide on the basis of dignity can now be made clearer.

1. Every individual human being is a member of a natural kind that has intrinsic Dignity.

2. When sick and dying, the attributed dignities of human beings come under profound assault.

3. There is a duty to build up, to the extent possible, the attributed dignities of dying human beings (P-IV).

4. Given the finite nature of human beings, this duty (P-IV) is imperfect. In fact, it is impossible to prevent, restore, or ameliorate all

aspects of the diminution in attributed dignities that illness and death bring upon human beings.

5. In such circumstances, one can never act with the specific intention-in-acting of destroying the human being who is suffering these attributed indignities as a means of relieving their burden, because this would undermine the intrinsic Dignity that gives force to the duty to build up attributed human dignities in the first place (P-VI).

6. This does not imply that one must do everything technologically possible to prolong the life of an individual human being. Intrinsic Dignity is a supreme value, but it is a finite value. This is because human beings are finite, and respect for the value of human beings cannot deny their finitude.

11. Counter-Arguments

How could a proponent of euthanasia or physician-assisted suicide, whether in Europe, North America, or anywhere else in the world respond to such an argument?

First, one could deny that being human confers intrinsic Dignity. One might say it is arrogant and 'speciesist' to claim that being human, in and of itself, confers special value. This sort of argument is raised by ethicists such as Peter Singer.[17] But one must be careful to note that my argument is that *all* natural kinds have intrinsic value, not just the human natural kind. Singer privileges individual entities that can feel pain, arguing that this property alone makes something worthy of moral consideration.[18] However, this leads to at least two sorts of serious problems that he considers consequences of practical ethics rather than *reductio ad absurdam* refutations of his theory. First, on Singer's view we seem then to have no moral responsibilities (or at best only symbolic ones) towards human beings that cannot feel pain, such as those in permanent coma. Second, we seem

---

[17] P. SINGER, *Practical Ethics*, 2nd ed., New York, Cambridge University Press, 1993, pp. 55-82, pp. 274-276.

[18] *Ibid.*, pp. 56-58. Singer quotes Bentham's famous lines, "The question is not *Can they reason? Nor Can they talk? but Can they suffer?*" and argues that nothing but sentience qualifies for making something an object of moral concern.

to have no moral responsibility towards stars or plants except as they serve the interests of sentient beings, thereby endangering the possibility of a serious environmental ethics. My claim is that intrinsic Dignity is simply the name we give to the highest level in a hierarchy of intrinsic values that includes all natural kinds. Which theory is the exclusionary and prejudiced one? Singer's theory excludes plants and stars and the comatose from moral consideration. Mine does not. Which is the more impoverished theory of ethics — one based on the duties that human beings have to themselves, each other, and to the universe of value by virtue of the fact that they are members of a natural kind possessed of intrinsic Dignity, or a theory that bases all of ethics on the meagre (and exclusionary) premise that feeling pain is a bad thing?

Perhaps one might argue that the fact that my theory of intrinsic Dignity is a threshold concept makes it morally suspect because it functions as a type of exclusionary club. Perhaps it is 'speciesist' to insist that the intrinsic value of some natural kinds is in any way special. Wouldn't it be best to consider the intrinsic values of all natural kinds to be arranged along a more or less continuous spectrum? On this view, our moral obligations towards each natural kind would simply be relative to that natural kind's place in this hierarchy. There are several problems with this view, however. First, I agree that there is a continuum of intrinsic value among natural kinds. However, my view is based upon a richer notion of value. It seems suspiciously narrow to count the value of something in isolation from its relationships to other things and its value within the ecosystem. On my view, the value of each natural kind depends upon what kind of thing it is, and the kind of thing it is is embedded in a network of ecological relationships. Second, regardless of whether one accepts my richer notion of the value of a natural kind, it is just *obvious* that the nature of the human natural kind and its place within the ecosystem gives it the highest level along such a putative continuum of intrinsic value. If so, then human beings would just be the sole known natural kind at the top of a continuous scale of the intrinsic value of natural kinds. If one were to refrain as a matter of taste or for some other reason from calling this highest level of intrinsic value 'intrinsic Dignity', it would not matter functionally with respect to such questions as how one ought to treat human beings. All this counterargument could accomplish would be the creation a different label without making a moral difference. One would still treat all human beings as members of a natural kind that has the highest known intrinsic value, but refrain from calling that value intrinsic Dignity. Third, I define intrinsic Dignity as that level of intrinsic value that belongs to *any* natural kind that meets a threshold set of defining characteristic features and dispositional predicates. If this is how one defines it, then other natural kinds might arguably belong. Then one is not at all guilty of speciesism but in fact making the best possible case against an arbitrarily exclusive definition of intrinsic Dignity.

Still another form of this counterargument might be that there is no such thing as a continuum of intrinsic value — that intrinsic value is equal across all natural kinds and arises only from the bare fact of existence. In other words, one might grant that there is such a thing as intrinsic value, but assert that it is trivial and only means that every natural kind that exists has value independent of a valuer merely because it exists. A corollary of this position would be that any other value is attributed by a valuer, and that it is only this attributed value that differs between natural kinds. Of course, this would render the universe rather flat. The field of intrinsic value would be a pure white field. It would suggest that the respect that I owe to a human being qua human being is equivalent to the respect that I owe to an *E. coli* bacterium qua *E. coli* bacterium. The notion that the complexity, rationality, creativity, moral agency, etc. that are distinctive about the human natural kind do not entail a value for the human natural kind that in and of itself is more valuable than that of the natural kind, *E. coli*, seems farfetched. Further, on this line of argument, even making a statement that one natural kind is more complex than another becomes morally suspect. The very notion that evaluation is possible implies that there are differences in value to be evaluated. Grains of sand, on my account, do have intrinsic value. But it seems farfetched to say that this intrinsic value is exactly equal to that of a human being.

But perhaps this last objection really amounts to a denial that there is such a thing as intrinsic value. The notion that nothing has value except from the perspective of a valuer suggests the famous view of Protagoras that "Man is the measure of all things".[19] But certainly there can be no more anthropocentric view of the universe than this;

[19] This fragment comes from his book, *On Truth*. The exact quote (in English translation) is, "Of all things the measure is man: of existing things, that they exist; of nonexistent things, that they do not exist." J.M. ROBINSON, *An Introduction to Early*

no grosser form of speciesism than the view that no species has value except that conferred upon it by human evaluation. Obviously, human beings attribute value to many things. But the notion that a thing has intrinsic value does not preclude the possibility that human beings might attribute other values to that thing. Conversely, the fact that value might be attributed to a thing by a human valuer does not preclude the logical possibility that it might also have intrinsic value.

The view that nothing has intrinsic value is precisely the view that environmental ethicists are trying to counter. But other problems arise in ethics without a theory of intrinsic value. In human interaction, the possibility of ethics is radically threatened by such a position. If there is no reason one must respect the interests of a person, then that person has no moral claims on anyone else, and no protection. Even an intersubjective attribution of intrinsic value to a person in an 'as if' construction would not be a sustainable way out of this problem. If one were to build an ethic upon the premise that, "We should all act as if there were an intrinsic value to being human and act accordingly even though, enlightened by philosophy, we know that there really is no intrinsic value to anything," one would still be left with the problem of having to give a reason to behave in such an 'as if' fashion. This leads to the convoluted conundrum that deception and/or self-deception is a basis for morality, still leaves one open to the arbitrary whims of whoever's preferences are eventually codified as the 'as if' true moral precepts, and leaves all persons constantly susceptible to arbitrary changes in these precepts.[20] Ultimately, if one is to be concerned about the interests of a person, this must be founded upon a respect for some sort of value inherent in the person whose interests they are. This is the value I have called intrinsic Dignity.

Another form of objection might be to deny that all human beings have intrinsic Dignity, and to argue that intrinsic Dignity is only a feature of a class within the human natural kind, the class of persons. This is a very familiar argument. While the exact words might differ, in various forms, one hears it argued that *persons* have intrinsic Dignity, but that not all human beings are persons. Therefore it is

Greek Philosophy, Boston, Houghton Mifflin, 1968, pp. 245. The precise meaning is far from obvious, and I am using it here in one possible sense.

[20] J.A. RIST, *Real Ethics: Rethinking the Foundations of Morality*, Cambridge, Cambridge University Press, 2002, pp. 20-24.

morally permissible to euthanize or assist in the suicide of human beings who have lost their personhood.

On the theory I have presented, the problem with this line of argument is that truly intrinsic value belongs to natural kinds, not to classes of individuals, whether the individuals under consideration are within one natural kind or are individuals across different natural kinds. 'Person', as the term is used in these arguments, is not a natural kind. Person refers to a class. In the standard form of this argument, the author provides a list of predicates to define the class. Some human beings are in the class, and some are not, depending upon whether all of the necessary and sufficient characteristics of the class *person* can be predicated of them. Some commentators in this school might quibble about how much rationality or self-control or memory an individual must have in order to be considered a member of the class. But all theories of personhood used in these arguments depend upon the notion that 'person' denotes a class.

As I argued above, however, intrinsic value belongs to natural kinds, not classes. The intrinsic Dignity of a demented human being, on my theory, is the same as the intrinsic Dignity of a philosopher-king. The attributed dignities of the two may differ drastically. There may be a moral mandate to do more to build up the attributed dignities of the demented patient. But arguments about whether the demented patient is a person are moot with respect to intrinsic Dignity. Person denotes a class. Intrinsic Dignity, like any intrinsic value, belongs to natural kinds, not classes.

Natural kinds have law-like features or dispositional predicates that are characteristic of a typical member of that natural kind. Confusion may arise because the features and dispositional predicates that define the human natural kind overlap substantially with the predicates that are used to define the class of persons. Some individual members of the human natural kind do not express the characteristics that are typical of the human natural kind. Many of these failures to express species-typical characteristics constitute illnesses. One might argue that some ill individuals cease to be persons, but this does not imply that they thereby cease to be members of the human natural kind. If intrinsic value belongs to things by virtue of their being the kinds of things that they are, then intrinsic human Dignity belongs to human beings by virtue of the fact that they are human beings. While one might demur at saying that a human being who has lost all memory is still a person, one must acknowledge that such an individual remains a member of the human natural kind.[21]

Finally, one who objects to the argument against euthanasia and assisted suicide on the basis of intrinsic Dignity might grant that there is such a thing as intrinsic Dignity, but deny that this implies that one has an absolute moral obligation never to destroy an individual member of a natural kind possessed of such intrinsic Dignity. This objection could either be based upon a rejection of P-VI, or upon a rejection of the argument that euthanasia and assisted suicide violate P-VI (*i.e.*, that step 5 of the Dignity argument against euthanasia and assisted suicide is wrong).

P-VI states that, in carrying out PP-I-V, one ought never to act in such a way as directly to undermine the intrinsic Dignity that gives the other duties their binding force. Rejecting this principle would seem to be extremely difficult. It would seem to be a contradiction in practical reasoning to act in such a way as to undermine one's fundamental reason for acting. At a minimum, one ought to be coherent in one's practical reasoning. For instance, if the fundamental reason one engages in gardening is to enjoy the natural beauty of plants, and this is what justifies one's specific efforts to plant and to water and to weed, then it would seem inconsistent with that fundamental reason for acting to replace one's live garden with plastic flowers. Similarly, if intrinsic Dignity constitutes the fundamental reason that one is beneficent, non-maleficent, and just in one's actions (*i.e.*, if the reason one respects a human being's interests is that one respects the human being whose interests they are), then one ought not perform actions that undermine intrinsic Dignity.

So, the only coherent form of this counterargument must be that euthanasia and assisted suicide do not undermine intrinsic Dignity, and that these acts may even be the highest possible expressions of respect for the intrinsic Dignity of human beings. The impressive

---

[21] One way of understanding the classical definition of a person from Boethius as "an individual substance of a rational nature," is that it treats the concept of person as an individual member of a class of natural kinds of which rationality is a typical characteristic, rather than the name of the simple class of individuals of whom rationality can be predicated (*De persona et duabus naturis* ch. 1, *Patrologia Latina* 64, 1343; quoted in Aquinas, *Summa Theologiae* I., q. 29, a1). D. WIGGINS, *Sameness and Substance*, pp. 149-189, distinguishes between being a person and being a member of the human natural kind, but accepts rationality as one of the law-like principles that define the human natural kind.

powers of reason, moral action, creativity, etc. that afford for the human natural kind the status of intrinsic Dignity may be so compromised or undermined by a disease or its treatment that, according to a familiar argument, the only way truly to respect the intrinsic Dignity of a patient is intentionally to bring about the patient's death through assisted suicide or euthanasia.

But this is a confused argument. First, as I argued above, if there is such a thing as intrinsic Dignity (and in this argument we are assuming that the objector agrees that there is), then it does not admit of degrees and belongs to all members of the natural kind. Thus, if a thing is a member of a natural kind that has intrinsic Dignity (or any other intrinsic value), it has that value so long as it is what it is, and can lose that value only if it changes into something else — for example, if a human being becomes a pile of ashes or a hydatid mole. Thus, there is really only one easy and common way that one may undermine this value among fellow human beings — that is by killing (or assisting in the killing of) another human being.[22]

Illness certainly attacks the attributed dignities of patients, and a patient's situation may on some occasions become so bad that it raises the question of whether there is such a thing as intrinsic Dignity. But the physical appearance of patients, their degree of independence, their social worth, their ability to make rational choices, and other features commonly associated with dignity are all *attributed* dignities. These *do* admit of degrees, and when they are diminished the attributed dignity of the patient is diminished. But if there is such a thing as intrinsic Dignity, then these attributed indignities cannot eliminate it, no matter how savage may be their effects upon the patient.

Second, it seems confused to suggest that one can restore or respect the intrinsic Dignity of something by intentionally bringing about its destruction. This is as hopelessly paradoxical as the alleged logic of the Vietnam War, "We had to destroy the village in order to save it." Thus, if one says, "The only way we could respect his intrinsic Dignity was to euthanize him," one is seriously confused. One's motive,

---

[22] This assumes that one cannot change a member of the human natural kind into a different natural kind other than through destruction and dissolution. Genetic engineering may soon make other changes possible. So, one day, geneticists may be charged with witchcraft if they can, for instance, change someone into a newt.

in such cases, is likely to put an end to the attributed indignities that the illness has visited upon the patient. That is what palliation does. But P-VI puts a limit on this palliative effort — that one cannot pursue palliation at all costs. If one's plan for palliation undermines the intrinsic Dignity that gives the moral imperative to palliate its binding force to begin with, then one has a duty of perfect moral obligation not to pursue this plan. P-IV commits one to palliate. Thus, analgesics, anti-emetics, anti-depressants and other palliative medications would all be morally indicated, but euthanasia and assisted suicide would not.

12. Further Objections

The discussion above might lead to the further objection that the position I am defending is 'vitalism' and would not permit the withholding and withdrawing of life-sustaining treatments, since these would bring about the death of the patient in many cases as readily as would euthanasia or assisted suicide. However, P-VI is carefully constructed so as not to commit one to this position. The adverb 'directly' refers to the intentional state of the agent. I take this to mean that one should never act with the specific intention in acting of undermining the intrinsic Dignity of a thing that has intrinsic Dignity by way of one's action. In the case of human beings, I have just established that this implies that one cannot set as one's intention in acting the bringing about of the death of a human being by way of one's action.

But propositions 4 and 6 of the argument against euthanasia and assisted suicide on the basis of intrinsic Dignity also take note of the important facts of human finitude and medical fallibility. Duties to build up attributed dignities are limited by the fact of death and the imperfections of the medical craft. These facts, together with P-VI, plus the philosophy of mind that grounds the distinction between intention and foresight[23], support the distinction between killing and

---

[23] See, for instance, A. DONAGAN, *Choice: The Essential Element in Human Action*, London, Routledge and Kegan Paul, 1989, pp. 40-41, p. 51; M. BRAND, *Intending and Acting*, Cambridge, MIT Press, 1984, pp. 94-97, pp. 122-126; M. BRATMAN, *Intention, Plans, and Practical Reason*, Cambridge, Harvard University Press, 1987, pp. 1-22, p. 37, p. 60, p. 141; J. SEARLE, *Intentionality: An Essay in the Philosophy of Mind*, New York, Cambridge University Press, 1983, pp. 7-10, pp. 35-36, pp. 103-105; D. GUSTAFSEN, *Intention and Agency*, Dordrecht, D. Reidel, 1986, p. 44, p. 68.

allowing to die. I have defended this distinction as philosophically valid.[24] At least in the United States, the Supreme Court has accepted this distinction as legally valid.[25] It remains a hotly contested point among philosophers in the United States, and space considerations will not permit me to pursue this line of argument further here.[26]

Finally, one cannot argue that allowing to die constitutes an undermining. Again, this raises significant issues far beyond the scope of this essay. However, a brief analogy may suffice to indicate the problems with this objection. Suppose that one accepts and deeply respects the value of a Giotto fresco, especially the frescoes in the Basilica of St. Francis in Assisi, Italy. After the terrible earthquake that shook Assisi in 1997, many of these frescoes were damaged. Some were fractured into so many hundreds and thousands of pieces that they would be almost impossible to re-assemble. Still, one might think of commissioning thousands of artists and art historians, paying them handsomely over decades, to piece these most severely damaged frescoes together. It would not, however, be unthinkable or disrespectful of Giotto or of medieval art or of St. Francis himself if one were to say that despite the value one recognizes in a Giotto fresco that one would not heroically work to undertake such a project and would accept the fact that this Giotto fresco had passed from the world. Nonetheless, if several *putti* at the corners of a severely damaged fresco survived the earthquake, and these parts were, in fact, all that remained of the fresco, one *would* consider it disrespectful of the work of art, the artist, the religious meaning of the place, etc. if someone were to take a sledgehammer and were to destroy what remained of the fresco under the pretext that it was so damaged that it was just no longer what it had been. "Allowing the fresco to die" would not seem to undermine one's respect for its value, while "killing" it *would* seem to undermine one's respect for its value. Analogously, the same could be said of our treatment of human beings at the end of life.

---

[24] D.P. SULMASY, 'Killing and allowing to die: Another look' in *Journal of Law, Medicine and Ethics* 26(1998), pp. 55-64; ID., *Killing and Allowing to Die*, Ph.D. Dissertation, Georgetown University, 1995.

[25] WASHINGTON V. GLUCKSBURG, 117 S. Ct. 2258 (1997); VACCO V. QUILL, 117 S. Ct. 2293 (1997).

[26] R. DWORKIN et al., 'Assisted Suicide: The Philosopher's Brief' in *New York Review of Books*, 27 March 1997, pp. 41-47.

Conclusion

Arguments on both sides of the debate about euthanasia and assisted suicide, on both sides of the Atlantic, frequently invoke the word 'dignity'. The word has proven conceptually important and morally powerful, but persistently vague in its meaning. In this essay I have tried to fit the word 'dignity' into a larger theory of value, distinguishing first between attributed and intrinsic values. I further subdivided attributed values into instrumental and non-instrumental, and identified a subset of non-instrumental attributed values called 'attributed dignities'. I divided intrinsic values into simple intrinsic values and intrinsic Dignity, the latter reserved for the intrinsic value of the highest levels of entities in the world, including (perhaps exclusively) human beings. I also showed that the concept of intrinsic value required a notion of natural kinds, and that this value belongs to all individual members of a given natural kind by virtue of these things being what they are. Whether in the Scottish highlands or the low countries of Belgium and the Netherlands, arguments favouring assisted suicide and euthanasia seem to make use of the word 'dignity' exclusively in the sense I have called 'attributed dignities'. The argument against euthanasia and assisted suicide is made exclusively on the basis of intrinsic Dignity. I explicated and defended this argument by showing that the potential counterarguments of those who favour euthanasia and assisted suicide would entail either that they give up their arguments in favour of these practices or give up the notion that there is such a thing as intrinsic Dignity. Giving up the notion of intrinsic Dignity, however, a notion that is deeply embedded in the Universal Declaration on Human Rights, and the European Convention on Human Rights and Biomedicine, would have dire consequences, at the very least, for the notions of civil rights, international law, and environmental ethics.

But the logical consequences of giving up the idea of intrinsic Dignity seem even greater. In denying the idea of intrinsic Dignity, one might be forced to give up on the notion of morality itself. This may help to explain Wittgenstein's observation that, "*Wenn der Selbstmord erlaubt ist, dann ist alles erlaubt*".[27] With so much at stake, it is no wonder that the legalization of euthanasia and assisted suicide have

---

[27] L. WITTGENSTEIN, *Notebooks, 1914-1916*, (ed. G.H. VON WRIGHT & G.E. ANSCOMBE, transl. G.E. ANSCOMBE), Chicago, University of Chicago Press, 1979, p. 91.

proven so profoundly controversial. One can only hope that the people and governments of the Low Countries will realize that they have been mistaken in their moral views on this matter, and that other nations and peoples will not repeat their mistake.

References

AMES, P., 'Belgian bishops condemn Parliament approval of Euthanasia Bill' in *Associated Press Worldstream*, International News, 17 May 2002.

AQUINAS, T., *Summa Theologiae*, Blackfriars Edition, New York, McGraw-Hill, 1964.

BRAND, M., *Intending and Acting*, Cambridge, MIT Press, 1984.

BRATMAN, M., *Intention, Plans, and Practical Reason*, Cambridge, Harvard University Press, 1987.

BRODY, B., *Identity and Essence*, Princeton, Princeton University Press, 1980.

COUNCIL OF EUROPE, *Convention for the Protection of Human Rights and Dignity of the Human Being with Regard to the Application of Biology and Medicine: Convention on Human Rights and Biomedicine*, ETS no.164, to be found at *http://conventions.coe.int/Treaty/EN/CadreListeTraites.htm*.

DONAGAN, A., *Choice: The Essential Element in Human Action*, London, Routledge and Kegan Paul, 1989.

DWORKIN, R., *Taking Rights Seriously*, Cambridge, Harvard University Press, 1977.

DWORKIN, R., T. NAGEL, R. NOZICK, J. RAWLS, T. SCANLON & J. JARVIS THOMSON, 'Assisted Suicide: The Philosopher's Brief' in *New York Review of Books*, 27 March 1997, pp. 41-47.

GUSTAFSEN, D., *Intention and Agency*, Dordrecht, D. Reidel, 1986.

KANT, I., *Groundwork for the Metaphysics of Morals* (transl. J.W. ELLINGTON), Indianapolis, Hackett, 1981.

KANT, I., 'The Metaphysics of Morals, Part II: The Metaphysical Principles of Virtue' in *Ethical Philosophy*, (transl. J.W. ELLINGTON), Indianapolis, Hackett, 1983.

KNICKERBOCKER, B., 'Latest showdown over assisted suicide' in *The Christian Science Monitor*, 15 November 2001, p. 3.

LEMOS, N.M., 'Value' in R. AUDI (ed.), *The Cambridge Dictionary of Philosophy*, New York, Cambridge University Press, 1995, pp. 829-830.

LISSKA, A.J., *Aquinas' Theory of Natural Law: An Analytic Reconstruction*. Oxford, Clarendon Press, 1996.

NORDENFELT, L., 'Dignity and the Elderly.' Abstract presented at the XVIth European Conference on Philosophy of Medicine and Health Care, Malta, 23 August 2002.

RIST, J.A., *Real Ethics: Rethinking the Foundations of Morality*. Cambridge, Cambridge University Press, 2002.

ROBINSON, J.M., *An Introduction to Early Greek Philosophy*, Boston, Houghton Mifflin, 1968.

ROLSTON, J. III., *Environmental Ethics*, Philadelphia, Temple University Press, 1988.

SEARLE, J., *Intentionality: An Essay in the Philosophy of Mind*, New York, Cambridge University Press, 1983.

SINGER, P., *Practical Ethics*, 2nd ed., New York, Cambridge University Press, 1993, pp. 274-276.

SULMASY, D.P., 'Death and human dignity' in *Linacre Quarterly* 61(1994), pp. 27-36.

SULMASY, D.P., *Killing and Allowing to Die*, Ph.D. dissertation, Georgetown University, 1995.

SULMASY, D.P., 'Death with dignity: What does it mean?' in *Josephinum Journal of Theology* 4(1997), pp. 13-23.

SULMASY, D.P., 'Killing and allowing to die: AnotherlLook' in *Journal of Law, Medicine and Ethics* 26(1998), pp. 55-64.

SULMASY, D.P. 'Healing the Dying: Spiritual Issues in the Care of the Dying' in J. KISSEL & D.C. THOMASMA, *The Health Professional as Friend and Healer*, Washington DC, Georgetown University Press, 2000, pp. 188-197.

UNITED NATIONS, *Universal Declaration of Human Rights*, to be found at *http://www.un.org/Overview/rights.html*.

VACCO V. QUILL, 117 S. Ct. 2293 (1997).

VELLEMAN, J.D., 'A right to self-termination?' in *Ethics* 109(1999), pp. 605-628.

WASHINGTON V. GLUCKSBURG, 117 S. Ct. 2258 (1997).

WIGGINS, D., *Sameness and Substance*, Cambridge, Harvard University Press, 1980.

WITTGENSTEIN, L., *Notebooks, 1914-1916*, (ed. G.H. von Wright & G. E. Anscombe, transl. G.E. Anscombe), Chicago, University of Chicago Press, 1979.

THE SANCTITY OF AUTONOMY?
TRANSCENDING THE OPPOSITION BETWEEN
A QUALITY OF LIFE AND A SANCTITY
OF LIFE ETHIC

Tom Meulenbergs & Paul Schotsmans

Introduction

The Belgian and Dutch Euthanasia Acts both reflect in their own way
the public and political debate on end-of-life decision making in
which notions such as the dignity of the human person and respect
for the patient's autonomous wishes play a pivotal role. In this contribution, we go into more fundamental issues which arise on the
horizon of discussions on end-of-life decision making and, specifically, of debates on the desirability of a legal regulation of euthanasia. First, we will analyse what kind of notion of autonomy operates
in these discussions and lay bare its problematic nature. This analysis will provide us with a clarifying framework for the sanctity versus quality of life debate. The predominant influence of the principle of respect for autonomy has strong implications for every
medical-ethical debate where the patient is involved as one of the
stakeholders. As far as the euthanasia discussion is concerned, the
radical understanding of the principle of respect for autonomy res-
onates in the quality-of-life approach. After a first look at the opposing positions (quality versus sanctity of life), we will confront these
two ethics of life in an attempt to overcome the classic deadlock
between them. More specifically, we will argue the position that in
Christian ethics an integration of the so-called two ethics of life is
not beyond reach. Hereby, our appreciation of the principle of
respect for autonomy will be of significant importance for the proposed anthropological interpretation of the notions of 'sanctity' and
'quality'.

1. Autonomy and only Autonomy

The central axis of both the Belgian and Dutch Euthanasia Act is the patient's right to self-determination, based on the principle of respect for autonomy that has had a predominant influence in recent medical-ethical discussions. A great deal of this 'success' goes back to the triumph of 'principlism', a school of thought which has its main theoretical foundations in the *Principles of Biomedical Ethics* and that is built upon four clusters of principles that guide medical actions (the principles of respect for autonomy, nonmaleficence, beneficence and justice).[1] In Hippocratic medicine, the principles of nonmaleficence and beneficence played key roles but in the contemporary health care setting autonomy has become the most important principle. When different principles are conflicting, it is often the principle of autonomy that overrides the other principles. The special status of the principle of autonomy is not only reflected in the discussions about euthanasia but also lays the foundation for the development of informed consent in the context of human experimentation, the right to refuse treatment, the right to abortion and so on. This is especially the case in the Anglo-American context where a strong tradition of personal liberties and privacy rights exists. During the last decades, legal cases have emphasised the central importance of respect for autonomy and the right to self-determination.[2] Yet, the proponents of the principlist approach have argued several times that the principle of respect for autonomy is an important moral limit but, nevertheless, is limited itself in scope and weight.[3]

The four principles approach is very much a product of its age and its culture. Beauchamp and Childress themselves indicate that "these principles initially derive from considered judgments in the common

---

[1] The very beginning of principlism can be traced back to *the National Commission for the Protection of Human Subjects of Biomedical and Behavioral Research*, installed in accordance to the U.S. National Research Act (1974). The commission's work resulted in the *Belmont Report*, the first principlist document (published in 1976 and officially promulgated by the U.S. Congress in 1978). Tom Beauchamp participated as a consultant in a draft of the *Belmont Report*.

[2] See e.g. ROE V. WADE. 410 U.S. 113, 93 S. Ct. 705, 35 L. Ed. 2d 147 (1973): the U.S. Supreme Court acknowledged a woman's personal right to abortion as based on the constitutional right to privacy; also SUPERINTENDENT OF BELCHERTOWN STATE SCHOOL V. SAIKEWICZ. 370 N.E.2d 417 (Massachusetts 1977): the court based the right to refuse treatment on the principle of self-determination.

[3] J.F. CHILDRESS, 'The place of autonomy in bioethics' in *Hastings Center Report* 20 (1990), pp.12-17.

morality and medical traditions".[4] Therefore, one can hardly imagine that the worship of the individual and its liberties would be absent in a set of principles especially designed to guide medical-ethical decision making. We believe, however, that it is strictly necessary to confront this ethic with some theoretical reflections upon the nature of the principle of respect for autonomy as well as on its ontological presumptions.

As one of the most basic ethical principles, respect for autonomy forbids the reduction of human beings to merely instruments. Immanuel Kant, in his *Grundlegung zur Metaphysik der Sitten* (1785) and subsequently in the *Kritik der Praktischen Vernunft* (1788), elaborated this account of respect for autonomy, which is condensed in the second formulation of the categorical imperative: "Treat others and oneself, never merely as a means, but always at the same time as an end in himself."[5] Contemporary authors in medical ethics often build their arguments upon Kant's philosophy. In their analysis of the principle of respect for autonomy Beauchamp and Childress refer to Kant who "argued that respect for autonomy flows from the recognition that all persons have unconditional worth, each having the capacity to determine his or her own destiny".[6] However, the question arises whether the modern principle of respect for patient autonomy is fully compatible with the Kantian notion of autonomy. We believe these two concepts are very different. A closer look at the sense of 'autonomy' in Kant's philosophy uncovers the fundamental difference between Kant's notion of autonomy and the principle of respect for patient autonomy used in contemporary medical-ethical debate. For Kant, the principle of autonomy is not a matter of willfulness but it is "to choose only in such a way that the maxims of your choice are also included as universal law in the same volition".[7] Thus, the Kantian notion of autonomy is far from

---

[4] T.L. BEAUCHAMP & J.F. CHILDRESS, *Principles of Biomedical Ethics*, New York, Oxford University Press, 2001, p.23.

[5] "Handle so, daß du die Menschheit, sowohl in deiner Person, als in der Person eines jeden andern, jederzeit zugleich als Zweck, niemals bloß als Mittel brauchest." in I. KANT, *Grundlegung zur Metaphysik der Sitten*, in W. WEISCHEDEL (ed.), *Immanuel Kant: Werke in sechs Bänden*, Band IV, Darmstadt, Wissenschaftliche Buchgesellschaft, 1983, p. 61.

[6] T.L. BEAUCHAMP & J.F. CHILDRESS, *Principles of Biomedical Ethics*, p. 63-64.

[7] "Nicht anders zu wählen, als so, daß die Maximen seiner Wahl in demselben Wollen zugleich als allgemeines Gesetz mit begriffen sein". in I. KANT, *Grundlegung zur Metaphysik der Sitten*, pp. 74-75.

the absolute principle of respect for patient autonomy which defends autonomous choice merely because it is the expression of the individual's needs or desires. Kant characterises the autonomous person as someone who makes choices based on impersonal, general laws and not by reason of appeal to the person's own needs or desires. The fundamental divergence between Kant's understanding of autonomy and the emphasis on patient autonomy in recent discussions can be illustrated by the different valuation of euthanasia. For Kant, there is no such thing as the right to end one's life. In his *Metaphysik der Sitten*, he clearly states that the maxim one should end one's life when it becomes excruciating is not universalisable and thus cannot be a legitimate moral maxim: "If adversity and hopeless grief have quite taken away the taste for life; if an unfortunate man (...) wishes for death and yet preserves his life without loving it, not from inclination or fear but from duty, then his maxim has moral content."[8] In recent discussions on physician-assisted suicide and voluntary active euthanasia, on the other hand, it is argued that there are sufficient grounds to justify assisted suicide and mercy killing. The main ground for justification is nearly always the principle of respect for autonomy. In cases of a genuine autonomous choice to die, i.e. an intentional choice based on understanding and without controlling influences, the individual's choice outweighs every other possible consideration. So contemporary respect for patient autonomy accepts every choice, if autonomous, as morally compelling whereas Kant restricts this qualification to choices based on pure reason. It seems to us that defenders of the modern principle of patient autonomy cannot fairly invoke Kant's philosophy in their defence of an absolute conception of patient autonomy for the simple reason that their understanding of autonomy is fundamentally different from Kant's principle of autonomy.

We believe that the contemporary understanding of the principle of respect for autonomy is more closely related to John Stuart Mill's conception of autonomy as described in *On Liberty*. Mill asserts that "the only freedom which deserves the name, is that of pursuing our

---

[8] "(...) wenn Widerwärtigkeiten und hoffnungsloser Gram den Geschmack am Leben gänzlich weggenommen haben; wenn der Unglückliche (...) den Tod wünscht, und sein Leben doch erhält, ohne es zu lieben, nicht aus Neigung, oder Furcht, sondern aus Pflicht: alsdenn hat seine Maxime einen moralischen Gehalt." in *Ibid.*, p. 23.

own good in our own way, so long as we do not attempt to deprive others of theirs, or impede their efforts to obtain it".[9] The Millian notion of autonomy — or freedom as autonomy — is totally different from the Kantian interpretation. John Stuart Mill does not restrict the label 'autonomous' to choices made on the basis of pure reason. Everyone is free to determine his own fate as long as the rights of others are not violated. In consequence, this Millian perspective on the autonomy argument rules out the terminal illness requirement for physician-assisted death. Euthanasia is, thus, open to terminal and nonterminal patients who have freely decided that their lives are no longer worth living.[10] The main criterion for autonomy is the fact that one pursues his good in his own way and hereby we believe the advocates of patient autonomy have a supportive ally in Mill but not in Kant.

2. Two remarks

In contemporary bioethical discussions, it is this Millian or, in more general terms, the libertarian view of autonomy which is promoted. This has not always been the case. During the 1960s and 70s, the principle of respect for autonomy has gained in power because of the traditional paternalistic Hippocratic ethic. For centuries, medical paternalism was common practice and physicians treated their patients in order to benefit them but mostly without the real consent of the patients themselves. It was the introduction of the principle of respect for patient autonomy that marked a new era in medicine. In this setting, autonomy had only a limited role, designed to fulfil the transient, narrow purpose of challenging the physician's paternalism.[11] The antithesis of autonomy and beneficence as well as the strained relation between the beneficent physician and the self-aware patient were the actual sources of the 'early meaning' of the principle of respect for patient autonomy.

---

[9] J.S. MILL, *On Liberty and Other Essays*, Oxford, Oxford University Press, 1998, p. 17.

[10] M. GUNDERSON & P.J. MAYO, 'Restricting physician-assisted death to the Terminally Ill' in *Hastings Center Report* 30(2000)5, pp. 18-19.

[11] R.M. VEATCH, 'Autonomy's temporary triumph' in *Hastings Center Report* 14(1984)5, pp. 38-40.

Since the early stages of the field of bioethics in the 1970s, the scope and the meaning of the principle of autonomy has, however, shifted away from a relational account of autonomy to an uncompromising veneration of personal autonomy. For talk of autonomy not to be meaningless or irrelevant in this new mindset, the human person has to have, in principle, the potential to take up this right to self-determination. This capability consists of the ontological premises of the human self as embodied in the non-relativist account of personal autonomy: the self is unencumbered, free to query and discard every particular relationship. The human person is depicted as completely detached from his social situation and cannot be determined by his intersubjectivity. Thus, every human person finds himself disconnected from others and from his own nature. As such, relational responsibility and alienation are necessarily related. This becomes, for example, perfectly clear in the discussion on care for the dying revealed in the euthanasia movement. There is in the autonomy approach no sound argument to prohibit a person, freed from all social or ontological bindings, to decide that he wants to die. If all human persons are fundamentally detached from each other, people should not consider their relational responsibilities when, for example, writing advance directives with a clear euthanasia component. The sheer fact that it is the person's own choice is considered the sole right-making characteristic of this choice. To the degree this liberal anthropology and the ontological premises involved are accurate, an autonomy-centred ethics could serve us well. However, since the advocates of autonomy leave the impression that a patient is always in a sort of Olympian control, we believe this portrayal of the individual is rather unreal, especially when we are dealing with the desperately ill and the dying. The idea that illness is irrelevant to someone's capacity — or obligation?[12] — to make his or her own choice neglects the influence illness has on people. The risk of the specific nature of the physician-patient relationship being disturbed or misunderstood because of the too individualistic and contractual approach clearly exists. This is affecting both the patient and the medical care.

---

[12] In the latest edition (2001) of their *Principles of Biomedical Ethics*, Beauchamp and Childress argue against the critique that they force choices on patients. According to these two authors, they defend a principle of respect for autonomy with a correlative *right* to choose and not a mandatory *duty* to choose. T.L. BEAUCHAMP & J.F. CHILDRESS, *Principles of Biomedical Ethics*, p. 61.

Secondly, an absolute defence of the principle of autonomy entails a number of undesirable consequences. By rejecting the possibility of intrinsic worth, liberals are confirming questionable tendencies of the modern self such as indifference and individual narcissism.[13] The assertion that there are no such things as universal intrinsic values implies the privatisation of all value judgements and, even, the decrease of public sphere. When every ethical appraisal is made part of the self-determination of the human self, one can ask the question whether there is not something more important at stake, that is to say the fading of public encounters where one can meet to discuss ideas and to confront personal considerations. The individualisation of ethical appraisal reduces the public debate to setting out limits to the scope of individual autonomy. Hence, we have no sincere interest in what appraisals others are making providing they are not interfering with our autonomy and our right to self-determination. This decrease of the public sphere entails major consequences. Some authors have clearly characterised this impact of decrease of the public sphere in terms of a loss of freedom, stability and plurality together with a sacrifice of objectivity and shared history.[14] There is a growing awareness that extending the claims of autonomy can undermine the social (e.g. families and civic institutions) and mental (e.g. processes of socialisation and moral development) infrastructure upon which social order, and hence the conditions for autonomy itself, rests.[15]

3. A Quality-of-Life Ethic as a Radical Defence of the Autonomy Principle[16]

There exists a clear link between, on the one hand, a radical quality-of-life approach and, on the other hand, the predominant influence

---

[13] H. DE DIJN, *Hoe overleven we de vrijheid? Modernisme, postmodernisme en het mystiek lichaam* [How can we survive liberty? Modernism, postmodernism and the mystic body], Kapellen, Pelckmans, 1993, pp. 78-79.

[14] See, for instance, Hannah Arendt's analysis of the decrease of public sphere in consequence of the rise of economic activities to the public realm in H. ARENDT, *The Human Condition*, Chicago, The University of Chicago Press, 1958.

[15] W. GAYLIN, 'Worshiping autonomy' in *Hastings Center Report* 26(1996)6, p. 45.

[16] See H. KUHSE, *The Sanctity-of-Life Doctrine in Medicine. A Critique*, Oxford, Oxford University Press, 1987. This book is one of the best introductions to this discussion. Helga Kuhse, an associate of Peter Singer, takes a clear position in favour of a radically autonomous and subjective Quality-of-life Doctrine.

of the principle of respect for autonomy in medical-ethical decision making. John Stuart Mill argued that the only legitimate basis on which the state may coerce the individual is to protect others. The individual's own good, whether physical or mental, is not a sufficient warrant for state intervention. Hence, Mill challenged, together with other British philosophers such as Jeremy Bentham and David Hume, the absolute prohibition of euthanasia as well as the negative approach towards suicide and infanticide. This is also the opinion of the *Royal Dutch Medical Association* (KNMG) when they suggest that the crucial question in euthanasia decisions is whether the patient wants to die on the basis of what he regards as unbearable suffering. Defenders of a quality-of-life approach share this view and believe that competently informed patients should be allowed to die when, from their point of view, life in a distressing or seriously debilitating condition is no longer worthwhile. Different patients will decide differently under similar circumstances because different patients have different goals and different values. An advocate of a quality-of-life ethic would suggest that these goals and values ought to be respected. The interpretation of quality of life is therefore a radical choice for the principle of autonomy as a dominant principle in bioethics. What is important and what should be protected at any cost is not merely life but the autonomy of the patient.

The original quality-of-life approach started from the question 'What is special about human life?' Two answers were posited. The first answer is typical for the sanctity-of-life approach: human life has sanctity simply because it is human life; that is, because it is the life of a member of the species *Homo Sapiens*. The second answer is typical for the quality-of-life approach: human life has special value because humans are self-aware, rational, autonomous, purposeful, moral beings, with hopes, ambitions, life purposes, ideals and so on. Any of these qualities, or a combination of them, could serve as a basis for a moral distinction between human beings and lettuce or chickens, for example. That such distinguishing qualities are needed is clear, for if value were based merely on life, rather than on one or more of the above characteristics, then every life, including that of the earthworm or lettuce, would be equally valuable.[17] However, one would not, according to

---

[17] This approach is apparent in the deontologically based *Animal Rights Movement* which asserts animals are considered as having rights because they are *subjects of life*.

this view, be able to argue that the lives of all members of the human species have special value; for example, the lives of the irreversible comatose, or the lives of the severely brain-damaged newly born infants. This second approach, then, does not give us a reason for preserving all human lives and cannot serve as the basis for the view that all human lives, irrespective of their quality or kind, are equally valuable.

The first answer, life has sanctity because it is human, covers all human beings by definition. Kuhse criticises this position and believes that the fact that a being belongs to the species *Homo Sapiens*, rather than to any other species, cannot tell us anything about the value of that being's life. In her opinion, the value of human life and the wrongness of taking it must not rest on *speciesism*. She is referring here to the view that human life has special value simply because it is human life.[18] Just as race or sex are not morally relevant in themselves, neither is species, following Kuhse. What is important is not that a patient is human and therefore should have his life sustained. Rather, we must ask questions about the quality and kind of life that the patient possesses. This approach is symbolic for the more utilitarian or consequentialist models in the ethical debate.

Kuhse starts with the assumption that conscious life has value because it enables a being to experience pleasurable states of consciousness. While the existence of pleasurable states is not the only value to which human life gives rise, it will be agreed, in her opinion, that it is at least a value that morality ought to take into account. She suggests clearly that life is not an intrinsic good, not a good in itself, but rather a means to achieve something else, for example, pleasurable states of consciousness. Therefore, if we are to agree that the value of life is not in life *qua* life (mere life), but rather life has its locus in the value it has for the individual concerned, then it would follow that life is not an unconditional good; rather, a good only insofar as it is of value to its possessor. This means that not all life is equally valuable, as the sanctity of life proponents suggest, nor is it always inviolable. Kuhse proposes a strong connection between the value of life and the interests of the being whose life it is. Life may

See T. REGAN, *The Case for Animal Rights*, Berkeley, University of California Press, 1983, especially pp. 243-248.

    [18] P. SINGER, *Practical Ethics*, Cambridge, Cambridge University Press, 1993.

be in a being's interests, or it may not, depending on what that life is like.

But when is a life, or death, in a patient's best interest, according to Kuhse? In order to answer this question, it is important to distinguish not only between different qualities of life (lives, for example, that are filled with unrelievable suffering and lives that allow for pleasure or happiness), but also between different kinds of lives. For example, differentiation can be made in the kinds of life experienced by normal adults in contrast to the kinds of life experienced by newly born infants and foetuses. In the context of prenatal testing procedures and the subsequent availability of abortions, she refers to a quality-of-life ethic that distinguishes between different kinds of life and associates the kinds of life to the wrongness of taking life. Referring to Michael Tooley, she reserves the term 'person' for those beings who are capable of understanding that they are continuing selves.[19] According to this view, neither human foetuses, human infants, human beings with severe mental retardation, nor humans with severe brain damage are persons. Consequently, it would not be directly wrong to take their lives. On the other hand, non-human animals, such as chimpanzees would, in Kuhse's view, have to take into account principles such as these. It would mean that the direct wrongness of killing lies not in taking life, but rather in overriding in a most profound way the interests, desires, and preferences of a person who does not want to die. This will have profound implications for decision-making in the practice of medicine.

The question is therefore no longer whether decisions to end human lives should sometimes be made; rather, the question is on what principle or principles these inevitable life and death decisions should be based. All patients capable of experiencing states of consciousness have an interest in well-being, that is, in freedom from pain, freedom from suffering, restoration of function, and so on. In addition, normal adult patients (persons) also have an interest in their own future, that is, in controlling and shaping their lives, and in acting as autonomous moral agents. In other words, Kuhse suggests that there are two main values to which human life gives rise: (1) pleasurable states of consciousness and (2) the value of autonomy or self-determination.

---

[19] M. TOOLEY, *Abortion and Infanticide*, Oxford, Clarendon Press, 1983.

4. Sanctity of Life

Few moral convictions are more deeply ingrained in the practice of medicine than the sanctity of life doctrine. In this context, sanctity of life means the sanctity of human life whereby all human life is in theory equally valuable and inviolable. Life refers to the bodily human life, meaning that life and death decisions must not be based on quality-of-life considerations. This doctrine has two basic characteristics: (1) inviolability and (2) the equal value of human life. The first characteristic, the inviolability of human life, implies that the sanctity of life doctrine prohibits the intentional termination of innocent human life, although not to be held in universal form. It prohibits 'doing' certain things to people rather than bringing about some results. It requires that we avoid intentionally taking life at all costs and not that we prevent death at all costs. There are two ways in which we can bring about death: to do something which results in someone's death and to fail to do something, as a result of which someone dies.

The second characteristic, the equal value of human life, indicates that the doctrine excludes both quality and kind of life as morally relevant factors when deciding whether or not to prolong a patient's life. All human lives are equal and worthy of the same protection, irrespective of their quality or kind. Considerations such as anticipated or actual limited potential of an individual are irrelevant and must not determine the decisions concerning medical care. Human life constitutes an irreducible value. The same effort must go into prolonging someone's life, regardless of whether the patient is irreversibly comatose or has a good chance of recovery. Conjoining these two basic characteristics, we clarify the prohibitory scope of the sanctity-of-life doctrine: "It is absolutely prohibited either to intentionally kill a patient or to intentionally let a patient die, and to base decisions relating to the prolongation or shortening of human life on considerations of its quality or kind."[20]

Regardless of how strongly the sanctity of life principle is integrated into the moral tradition, it does not impair the reality that there seems to be a consensus on 'letting die'. Supporters of the principle believe that the principle can be combined with a limited duty of life-preservation. They subscribe to a more nuanced version of the principle: "It is absolutely prohibited either intentionally to kill a patient or intentionally to let a patient die, and to base decisions

---

[20] H. KUHSE, *The Sanctity-of-Life Doctrine in Medicine*, p. 11.

relating to the prolongation or shortening of human life on considerations of its quality or kind; *it is, however, sometimes permissible to
refrain from preventing death.*"[21] This distinction between intentionally
killing a patient or letting die is however not always acknowledged.
The indistinctness of both concepts characterizes the Dutch debate
on euthanasia. For 35 years, do-not-resuscitate policies as well as
other non-treatment options were not present in the Dutch debate on
euthanasia.[22]

From the libertarian perspective on autonomy, however, one cannot fully understand what is meant by the notion 'sanctity of life', as,
in that perspective, one cannot accept shared intrinsic values. In the
liberal view, there are no goods which are valuable in themselves for
the reason that valuable goods are accustomed to fit the pattern of
individual choices, which are determined by rational preferences or
by merely biological needs. Hence, the worth of life depends exclusively on the individual's preferences. When the individual person
considers his life not as principle but merely as a means to pleasure,
he is fully entitled to take his own life in the absence of pleasure.
Consequently, life cannot be understood as having a universal intrinsic worth as implied by the notion of 'sanctity'.

5. A Deontological Remark from the 'Sanctity of Life' Doctrine[23]

John R. Connery, an advocate of the sanctity-of-life doctrine, considers the introduction of a quality-of-life consideration as radically new.
The question raised is: 'What effect does the quality of a patient's life
have on his duty to preserve it?' Can it be so low that it affects the
obligation to preserve this life even to the point of removing all treatment obligations? Connery refers to the traditional approach of
Roman Catholic moral theologians, who have admitted that the
obligation to preserve or to prolong life was not an absolute one but
rather a limited obligation. They discussed this duty and its limits in

---

[21] *Ibid.*, p. 23 (our italics).

[22] H. TEN HAVE, 'Euthanasia and the Power of Medicine' in D.C. THOMASMA *et al.*,
Asking To Die: Inside the Dutch Debate About Euthanasia, Dordrecht, Kluwer Academic
Publishers, 1998, p. 206.

[23] See J.R. CONNERY, 'Quality of Life' in J.J. WALTER & T.A. SHANNON (eds.), *Quality of Life: the New Medical Dilemma*, New York, Paulist Press, 1990, pp. 54-60.

terms of a distinction between so-called 'ordinary' and 'extraordinary' means. If means were excessively burdensome, or if they would not prolong life in any appreciable way, one could not impose an obligation on a person to use them. When a patient refused ordinary means, such a refusal was seen as intentional termination of life and, thus, negatively evaluated. This decision must be faced with greater frequency today than in the past, since there are ways and means of preserving life today that were simply not previously available. But, for Connery this basically does not challenge the sanctity-of-life approach.

Connery is aware of the fact that those who oppose quality-of-life considerations are classified pejoratively as 'vitalists'. This term may, however, only be appropriately applied to those who make life a supreme value to which everything else must yield and who hold, consequently, that all possible means to preserve it must be used. However, we clearly misuse the term if we apply it to every advocate of the sanctity-of-life doctrine. The majority of these in no way subscribe to the opinion that life must be preserved at all costs. They admit that there is a limit to the obligation to preserve life. They simply deny that this limit is based on quality of life as such.

It is Connery's opinion that moving the criterion from quality of treatment to quality of life as such is not just another step in the same direction. He construes it to be a quantum leap. In the past, quality of life was considered only in reference to means. Means might be categorised as burdensome or their application might be classified as quantitatively futile. In the present usage it would become the basic consideration. Even if it does not classify the means as burdensome or futile, it is appealed to in order to justify what is done or not done. According to Connery, this involves a whole new attitude toward this issue, one which also raises serious questions. "When quality of life is in itself the basic consideration, the entire approach is different. The intention is not to free the patient of the burden of using some means, but the burden (or the uselessness) of the life itself. The only way to achieve this goal is by the death of the patient. So when one forgoes means because of quality of life considerations in this sense, the intention is the death of the patient. In this respect it differs vastly from the traditional approach. In the traditional approach, death was an unintentional side-effect of forgoing the treatment. In the current use, it is the intention in forgoing the treatment. Put briefly, in the traditional approach, one was making a legitimate application of the principle of double effect. In the present approach, one of the conditions for the legitimate use of that principle is violated (the evil effect is intended), so no such justification is available."[24]

Connery sees an additional problem in the use of quality-of-life norms. No norm has been suggested that would clearly define the cases to which it would be applied or exclude those to which it would not apply. In other words, it would put us on a slippery slope with no braking power. This kind of norm, says Connery, would end up to be a menace to society because of its lack of precision. The fear of some that without the use of quality-of-life criteria we would be overwhelmed with people living in institutions at a very low level of existence is not realistic according to Connery: "My judgement is that many, if not most of the decisions that are made to withdraw treatment could be justified because burdensome means are involved. Many of the means in question, even if ordinary in a crisis situation, can become burdensome when used on a long term basis. If a judgement can be made that long term use will be required, such treatment may become optional. Certainly, death is the result in any event. But it is important that it should not result from the use of a criterion as objectionable and as open to abuse as quality of life."[25]

6. Sanctity and Quality of Life: an Integration in Christian Ethics?[26]

6.1 *A deeper analysis of both concepts*

Some Roman Catholic ethicists and physicians are convinced that quality-of-life judgements serve as just another step toward an inevitable slide down the slippery slope. Such a slide moves quickly toward the killing of those who are the most vulnerable in society, viz. the dying, the comatose, the handicapped and the incurably demented. In contrast, other Roman Catholic moral theologians argue that quality-of-life judgements are fully consistent with the substance of the longstanding Roman Catholic tradition on the distinction between the ordinary and extraordinary means of preserving

[24] *Ibid.*, p. 59.
[25] *Ibid.*, pp. 59-60.
[26] J.J. WALTER, 'The meaning and validity of quality of life judgments in contemporary Catholic medical ethics' in *Louvain Studies* 13(1988), pp. 195-208.

life. James Walter, for instance, attempts to locate and analyse a few of the definitional and ethical issues that are at stake in the discussion over the legitimacy of quality-of-life judgements. It should be clear that he uses the notion 'quality of life' in another meaning than the one present in the writings of Tooley, Singer and Kuhse. Indeed, a quantum leap remains between their approach and Walter's integration of quality-of-life concepts. The reason is simply that the consequentialist approach sanctifies the principle of autonomy rather than offering a valuable philosophical contribution which adds clarity to the dilemma's solution.

It is not altogether clear what the meaning of the word 'life' is. At least part of the ambiguity or confusion in the discussion results from not clearly distinguishing life as mere biological existence from life understood as embodied personal existence. For instance, anencephalic neonates or patients in a persistent vegetative state certainly have biological existence, but neither will ever experience personal existence as most of us understand that notion, i.e. life with sapient consciousness and personal freedom. By making this distinction, we can add clarity to our valuations of physical life (evaluative claims), to our duties in relation to this life, and to our limits in preserving mere biological existence (normative claims).

What the advancements in technology in medicine have done is to call into question the traditional goals of medicine. No doubt, medicine rightfully seeks to prevent death (especially untimely death), to alleviate pain and physical suffering, and to promote health. Walter would argue that these goals, important as they are, must be viewed as subordinate to the more encompassing goal of serving the *purposefulness* of personal existence. Physicians promote health, prevent death, perform surgery, and relieve pain in order that their patients might continue to pursue material, moral and spiritual values in some fashion that transcends physical life. Pain, disease, general ill health, and death either frustrate our desires to pursue these values or make it impossible to pursue them at all. As a consequence, when medicine can no longer promote these values for a patient, or when, by its interventions, medicine will place a patient in a condition that makes the pursuit of *purposefulness* too burdensome, then medicine has reached its limits on the basis of its own principal reasons for existence.

How then do we define quality of life? Because the word 'quality' is ambiguous, the entire phrase 'quality of life' is subject to expansion to include just about anything. Such is the case when one links the word 'quality', as is frequently done, to the idea of excellence. The meaning of the word will then be found only at the horizons of our imaginations and desires. If we pursue this idea, we will, no doubt, find it very difficult to identify objective criteria by which to assess these judgements. One's worst fears about quality-of-life judgements will be realised because all patients who cannot achieve the ideal excellent life will be put at risk. 'Quality' constituted in this manner will surely open the possibility of denying treatment to the handi-capped and the dying, and perhaps even permit vulnerable classes like these to be actively killed.

Another possibility is to define 'quality' as a property or an attribute of physical and/or personal life. Walter believes that the most authors who argue against quality-of-life judgements, and even some who argue for their validity, will define the term in this way.[27] There are a number of complex issues at stake once 'quality' is defined as a property or an attribute, but, since we are limited in space, we will analyse only two: (1) the evaluative status of physical life which does not possess the valued property, and (2) the origin of and the limits to our obligations to preserve biological life (normative status).

6.1.1 The evaluative status of life

What is it that we value about physical life? Do we value physical life in and for the sake of itself, or do we value life because of some prop-erty that life possesses, e.g. cognitive capacities, as Kuhse states? It is unfortunate, says Walter, that these questions have led some ethicists to frame the contemporary debate in terms of a quality-of-life ethic versus a sanctity-of-life ethic. He thinks that this entire discussion about the evaluative status of human life may be misplaced. Those who argue for sanctity-of-life ethic over and against a quality-of-life ethic, Connery for example, are aware that physical life is not an absolute value. On this point they are in total agreement with the proponents of the quality-of-life ethic. However, they maintain that those who support a quality-of-life ethic afford either no degrees or varying degrees of value to physical life contingent on the presence

---

[27] See Kuhse's definition of quality as (1) pleasurable states of consciousness and (2) the presence of autonomy (supra).

of some properties that life possesses. Such a view is intolerable for several reasons. In the first place, this view denies the equal worth and the equality of persons. Secondly, it denies that all lives are inherently valuable and so some lives can be truly not worth living if some valuable properties are not present. Thirdly, by adopting a bi-level anthropology that is committed to sustaining physical life only as an instrumental value, this position denies that human life is valued historically as body-spirit.

These authors conclude that a sanctity-of-life ethic is superior because it can affirm the equality of life on the grounds that physical life is truly a *bonum honestum* (a good or value in itself) and not a *bonum utile* (a useful or negotiable value that is dependent on some other intrinsically valuable property). Some argue for this position by philosophically valuing a theory of goods that are incommensurable and others argue for it theologically by valuing persons as created in the image of God.

At first sight, both arguments seem well taken. Therefore, it is necessary to further clarify the quality-of-life position. First, it is essential to distinguish clearly and consistently between physical or mere biological life and personal life (personhood). Without this important distinction, the opponents of quality-of-life judgements are prone to move back and forth between the value of biological life and the value of personhood, leading into further confusion.

Second, those who support quality-of-life judgements should state explicitly that physical life is indeed a value that is not conditioned on any property. Describing physical life as a conditional value has left opponents open to the criticisms noted above. Walter therefore suggests that it would be better to claim that physical life is a *bonum onticum*, that is, a true and real value, but by definition a created and therefore a limited good. By so arguing, he can now affirm that all physical lives are of equal ontic value and that all persons are of equal moral value.

Third, the word 'quality' does not and should not primarily refer to a property or attribute of life as the ultimate criterion for valuation. Rather, the quality that is at issue is "the quality *of the relationship* which exists between the medical condition of the patient, on the one hand, and the patient's ability to pursue life's goals and purposes understood as the values that transcend physical life, on the other".[28] If we understand the phrase to refer to the

---

[28] J.J. WALTER & T.A. SHANNON (eds.), *Quality of Life*, pp. 81-82.

quality of a relation and not to a quality of life itself, then the evaluative status of physical life is no longer a central issue in the debate.

6.1.2 The normative status of life

Those who are opposed to a quality-of-life ethic believe that such an ethic logically entails a moral judgement on the valued qualities of life. Since morally normative judgements are statements about our moral duties and their limits toward supporting and protecting life, these authors fear that life and death decisions will be made solely on the presence or absence of certain qualities (properties) that a patient's life possesses. The result would be that our duties toward protecting life, especially those whose lives are most vulnerable, would be seriously eroded in society. The response to this erosion would then be the arguing for a sanctity-of-life ethic.

To define 'quality' as a property of physical or personal life entails defining explicitly or implicitly that which is called 'the normatively human'. Normative moral theories are concerned with establishing standards for the moral evaluation of actions and a rationale for our moral obligations. The proponents of the sanctity-of-life ethic subscribe to either a rights or rule deontology and accuse those who adopt a quality-of-life ethic of grounding moral obligations in some form of personal or social consequentialism. In other words, in the sanctity-of-life ethic, the duty to preserve physical life is grounded either in the patient's right to life or in the rules that require respect for life, justice, or care for another.

Because physical life is not an absolute value, those who argue for a sanctity-of-life ethic admit that there are definite limits to our obligations to preserve life. As a matter of fact, several authors admit that these limits and/or exceptions to our duties are controlled by quality-of-life considerations that are embodied in the traditional Roman Catholic distinction between ordinary and extraordinary means of treatment. John Connery, for example, concedes that qualitative factors or contingent qualities of life, such as the pain associated with using a certain medical treatment or the burdens associated with the attainment of medical treatment, limit the duty to preserve life either on the part of the patient or on the part of health care providers. Thus, they argue that the distinction between morally obligatory means and extraordinary means that are not morally obligatory remains essentially valid and applicable today.

The crucial point is that the proponents of the sanctity-of-life ethic reject all quality-of-life factors. What they reject is the derivation of our duties from the presence of certain properties of physical or personal life at the level of normative theory, e.g. the capacity for human relationships. In other words, quality-of-life judgements function appropriately in this ethic as a way of limiting or making exceptions to our duties. They are judgements strictly circumscribed by an assessment of the benefits and burdens of medical treatment considered in itself and/or of those benefits and burdens that will accrue to the patient as a result of treatment. The judgements themselves are grounded on deontological considerations beforehand, e.g. the right to life or respect for life. Thus, as long as the equality of both physical life and personhood is assured at the evaluative and normative levels, this ethic does in fact recognise the relative importance of quality-of-life judgements in medical decision making.

The debate among contemporary Roman Catholic theologians over the validity of quality-of-life judgements in the medical context will be at a deadlock, says Walter, as long as the terms of the debate continue to revolve around two opposing types of ethics, viz. sanctity of life versus quality of life.

6.2. *An integration?*

A successful overcoming of the deadlock, but surely not the solution to all problems, will depend in part on the admission of the insights of the other's approach. In this section we want to offer an outline to support a synthesis in rather broad strokes. According to Walter, one of the items that often remains as a hidden agenda behind this debate concerns the goals and limits of medicine. He proposed that the central and over-arching end of medicine is "to promote and enhance the purposefulness of physical and personal life". On the one hand, such a proposal about the goal of medicine contributes little to the discussion surrounding the worth or value of physical or personal life. On the other hand, the proposal does address the *raison d'être* of medical interventions and its limits, and provides some insight into the general meaning of the terms 'benefits', 'burdens', and 'best interests' of a patient. Walter is convinced that quality-of-life judgements should not be construed as judgements about the value of either the physical or the personal. They are not concerned with assessing qualities or properties that, when present, make life itself valuable. Rather, "these judgements are evaluative and normative claims or assessments about the relation between the patient's medical condition and the patient's ability to pursue material, moral and spiritual values which transcend physical life but do not give that life its very meaning and worth".[29] As such, they specify the meaning of the terms 'benefit', 'burdens', and 'best interests' of a patient. Beyond that, they mark out the boundaries of medical interventions within a given historical and cultural situation.

Even though all physical life is of equal ontic worth and all personal life is of equal moral value, the quality of the relation between these lives and the pursuit of values is not equal. Inequality is due to a complex of multiple factors. These factors include, for instance, genetic endowment, personal lifestyles, and individual's nurturing, and accessibility of values in culture. Certain configurations of these factors afford some people the good fortune of attaining a high quality of life. Other individuals, regrettably, are not as fortunate, and they must live most of their lives pursuing life's purposes at a suboptimal level.

There are certain people, however, who have no discernible or minimal qualitative relation between their medical condition and the pursuit of values. A growing number of theologians have argued that to these people, society has no moral obligation to prolong their physical lives. As a consequence, all treatment, including artificial nutrition and hydration can be withdrawn from them. In the past, most if not all of these lives in such conditions would have been mercifully ended by the underlying pathology. In contrast, the interventions of modern medical technology have not been as merciful.

Walter responds to the preceding approach with two important considerations. First, none of the theologians proposing this view has accepted the active killing of patients. Second, this view does not fall into either a eudaemonistic or an exclusionary use of quality-of-life judgements. These theologians have not drawn a line at the upper limits of pursuing life's purposes (eudaemonistic use), but they have sought to establish the lowest possible limits of what reasonable people would judge bearable and acceptable vis-à-vis the qualitative relation under consideration. Furthermore, this position does not

---

[29] *Ibid.*, p. 84.

exclude those who fall below these limits from our ordinary moral obligation not to kill them or to care for them.

Duties and their limits to prolong life that bear on health-care professionals are correlative to the patient's obligations and their limits. When it is determined that a patient no longer has an obligation to prolong physical or personal life, then medical personnel will not exclude the patient from their obligation to offer treatment but will acquiesce to the limits of the patient's obligations. Thus, all other things being equal, when medicine can intervene to ameliorate the quality of the relation between the patient's condition and the pursuit of life's goals, then such an intervention can be considered a benefit to the patient and is in his/her best interests. On the other hand, when medical intervention can only be a burden to the life treated, then it is contrary to the best interests of the patient, it is harmful to the patient and medicine has reached its limits on the basis of its own reason for existence and thus should not intervene except to palliate or to comfort the patient. Futile treatment of this sort includes proposed intervention that can offer the patient no reasonable hope of pursuing life's purposes at all, that can only offer the patient a condition where the pursuit of life's purposes will be filled with profound frustration, or that produces anguish because of the energy needed to merely sustain physical life leads to utter neglect of these purposes.

What should be obvious is that quality-of-life judgements are concerned with what the Roman Catholic Church, in the *Declaration on Euthanasia* (1980) and the Encyclical *Evangelium Vitae* (1995), called the assessment of a due proportion between the benefits and the burdens. However, the proportionality referred to is not about the benefits and burdens of the treatment considered in themselves and apart from the patient; rather, the assessment is concerned with the proportionality of benefits and burdens (considered teleologically) that will affect the quality of the relation between the patient's medical condition and his/her pursuit of values. By adopting this view of quality-of-life judgements, it seems that the so-called two ethics of life are not two but really one.

7. A Plea for a Non-Absolutist Account of Autonomy

As with the opposition between a quality-of-life versus a sanctity-of-life ethic, we do not believe that a radical choice for one specific approach is beneficial in the debate between upholders of a non-relativist account of the principle of respect for autonomy and their critics. Rather, we think that there is need for an integration of the concerns of the advocates of patient autonomy on the one hand and the relational-personalistic view on the other hand. In clinical settings, autonomy is more an objective than an actual condition. The most basic fact is however the patient's vulnerability and endangered autonomy is just one of the many dimensions of this vulnerability. Therefore autonomy cannot be the only concern in medical-ethical decision making.

Furthermore, a principlist approach where respect for autonomy is the be-all and end-all of medical-ethical decision making, fails to give answers to all questions involved. It does not address the nature of human beings or the characteristics of human life. Neither does it make clear when human beings are being reduced to instruments. Therefore, we can agree with van Tongeren, that another approach is needed, different from the radical use of the principle of self-determination.[30] It demands that ethicists should pursue with great diligence all possible dimensions of reality instead of narrowing the discussion to merely rules, rights and duties and their justification and application. We must apply our abilities to understand moral possibilities, that is our moral sensitivity or sense.

We believe that a relational-personalistic view can make more sense for this understanding of our moral sensitivity than the liberal view of the unencumbered self. In providing a complete image of the human person, the relational-personalistic view avoids the one-sidedness of the absolutized autonomy-approach. It considers the human person as essentially decentralised without being alienated. A first mode of this *decentrement* consists of passivity at the core of the human self.[31] The source of the self is not placed in human subjectivity and, hence, made inaccessible for the human self. Thus, we are attached to something we cannot get away from but we cannot access either. Obviously, these considerations about the *decentrement*

---

[30] P.J.M. VAN TONGEREN, 'Ethical manipulations: An ethical evaluation of the debate surrounding genetic engineering' in *Human Gene Therapy* 2(1991), pp. 71-75.

[31] Visker illuminates the decentrement of the human subject in R. VISKER, *Truth and Singularity. Taking Foucault into Phenomenology*, Dordrecht, Kluwer Academic Publishers, 1999.

and the passivity at the core of the human self are apparent in Martin Heidegger's *Sein und Zeit* where he characterises the human condition as *Sorge*. To gain authenticity *Dasein* needs to be *entschlossen*. In his later work, Heidegger will put emphasis on a more passive responsiveness, i.e. *Gelassenheit*. We think this approach to the human self is an important counterpart of the human self depicted as self-determining. Evidently, the human person is not at all completely compelled by external forces or conditions exterior to the self. But, at the same time, we are aware of the fact that an overcharged appreciation of the principle of autonomy is based on a view of the human self which lacks this element of fundamental passivity in the heart of the human self, that is to say the fundamental inaccessibility of the human self. As, for example, oncologists regularly describe, patients cannot make up their mind. One moment, the patient is highly enthusiastic about the treatment when later on the day he or she does not want to recover at all. Thus, there is the patient's indecisiveness that brings about this ambivalent attitude towards curing. We believe this ambivalent behaviour, often met by general practitioners and medical specialists confronted with severely ill patients, can be interpreted as a reflection of certain movements within the essence of the patient that are for the patients themselves — and a fortiori for third parties such as proxies or medical staff — inaccessible.

Above and beyond this, there exists another, second, mode of *decentrement* of the human self concerning the intersubjectivity of the human person. A personalistic philosophy regards dedicating oneself to the other as a part of the process of self-discovery. The ethical task to love one's neighbour is our very essence. Intersubjectivity, as expressed in love, is rooted in the nature and createdness of humanity itself. I can only dedicate myself actively and consciously to my fellow human beings and to the world because I am structured, according to my essence itself, as a "being-for-the-other-than-myself".[32] However, every process of self-discovery is bound to be confronted with the boundaries correlated with the first mode of *decentrement*, the fundamental inaccessibility of the human self.

Anyway, these two modes of *decentrement* of the human self question also Kant's understanding of autonomy. As we have

---

[32] R. BURGGRAEVE, *Emmanuel Levinas. The Ethical Basis for a Humane Society*, Leuven, Acco, 1981.

described above, Kant sees the autonomous agent as someone who makes choices based on impersonal, general laws and not due to appeal to personal needs and desires. Both universality and rationality are important features of the Kantian notion of autonomy. The question arises if this understanding of autonomy does not have a blind spot for essential features of the human self other than the capacity for reason. Human autonomy, then, cannot be properly understood when there is only reference to men's rational faculties. In recent years, the failure of the rational and universal account is conceptualised in the ethics of care. According to Joan Tronto, Kant's portrayal of the human self with as main characteristics its detachment, its rational nature and universality constitutes one of the main boundaries that "exclude some ideas of morality from consideration".[33]

What do these two modes of *decentrement* of the human self bring about for the notions of 'quality' and 'sanctity'? In our view, they give emphasis to the importance of an axiological interpretation of the notions 'sanctity' and 'quality' of life. The first mode of *decentrement* can bring us toward a more moderate view of autonomy and self-determination; a view that takes account of the ontological fact that the human self is not as transparent and controllable as the advocates of autonomy suggest. Hereby, we do not reject the worth and the achievements of the principle of autonomy in the last decades. Quite the reverse, we are fully aware of the enormous impact the pledge for autonomy has had — and still should have — for our lives. We only want to acknowledge that every human person every so often runs into difficulties in determining himself due to this fundamental passivity at the core of his being. A second ground to reject the overpowering role some want autonomy to have has its origin in Judeo-Christianism. From this perspective, autonomy is a necessary condition for the fulfilment of creatural solidarity. Nevertheless, autonomy may neither have the first nor the last word since it exists thanks to creatural solidarity. The human autonomy we are required to respect, therefore, cannot result in an absolute dominion over one's own life but has to be understood in a broader framework that acknowledges both the intrapersonal limits and interpersonal boundaries to the sanctity of autonomy.

---

[33] J.C. TRONTO, *Moral Boundaries. A Political Argument for an Ethic of Care*, New York, Routledge, 1993, pp. 6-9.

References

ARENDT, H., *The Human Condition*, Chicago, The University of Chicago Press, 1958.

BEAUCHAMP, T.L. & J.F. CHILDRESS, *Principles of Biomedical Ethics*, New York, Oxford University Press, 2001.

BURGGRAEVE, R., *Emmanuel Levinas. The Ethical Basis for a Humane Society*, Leuven, Acco, 1981.

CHILDRESS, J.F., 'The place of autonomy in bioethics' in *Hastings Center Report* 20(1990), pp.12-17.

CONNERY, J.R., 'Quality of Life' in J.J. WALTER & T.A. SHANON (eds.), *Quality of Life: the New Medical Dilemma*, New York, Paulist Press, 1990, pp. 54-60.

DE DIJN, H. *Hoe overleven we de vrijheid? Modernisme, postmodernisme en het mystiek lichaam* [How can we survive liberty? Modernism, postmodernism and the mystic body], Kapellen, Pelckmans, 1993.

GAYLIN, W., 'Worshiping Autonomy' in *Hastings Center Report* 26(1996)6, pp. 43-45.

GUNDERSON, M. & P.J. MAYO, 'Restricting physician-assisted death to the terminally ill' in *Hastings Center Report* 30(2000)5, pp.17-23.

KANT, I., *Grundlegung zur Metaphysik der Sitten*, in W. WEISCHEDEL (ed.), *Immanuel Kant: Werke in sechs Bänden*, Band IV, Darmstadt, Wissenschaftliche Buchgesellschaft, 1983.

KUHSE, H., *The Sanctity-of-Life Doctrine in Medicine. A Critique*, Oxford, Oxford University Press, 1987.

MILL, J.S., *On Liberty and Other Essays*, Oxford, Oxford University Press, 1998.

REGAN, T., *The Case for Animal Rights*, Berkeley, University of California Press, 1983.

SINGER, P., *Practical Ethics*, Cambridge, Cambridge University Press, 1993.

TEN HAVE, H., 'Euthanasia and the Power of Medicine' in D.C. THOMASMA, T. KIMBROUGH-KUSHER, G.K. KIMSMA & C. CIESIELSKI-CARLUCCI, *Asking to Die: Inside the Dutch Debate About Euthanasia*, Dordrecht, Kluwer Academic Publishers, 1998, pp. 205-220.

TOOLEY, M., *Abortion and Infanticide*, Oxford, Clarendon Press, 1983.

TRONTO, J.C., *Moral Boundaries. A Political Argument for an Ethic of Care*, New York, Routledge, 1993.

MILL, J.S., *On Liberty and Other Essays*, Oxford, Oxford University Press, 1998

VAN TONGEREN, P.J.M., 'Ethical manipulations: An ethical evaluation of the debate surrounding genetic engineering' in *Human Gene Therapy* 2(1991), pp. 71-75.

VEATCH, R.M., 'Autonomy's temporary triumph' in *Hastings Center Report* 14(1984)5, pp. 38-40.

VISKER, R., *Truth and Singularity. Taking Foucault into Phenomenology*, Dordrecht, Kluwer Academic Publishers, 1999.
WALTER, J.J., 'The meaning and validity of quality of life judgments in contemporary Catholic medical ethics' in *Louvain Studies* 13(1988), pp. 195-208.

YOU SHALL NOT LET ANYONE DIE ALONE
RESPONSIBLE CARE FOR SUFFERING
AND DYING PEOPLE

Roger Burggraeve

Introduction

Current ideas in applied ethics regarding assistance for the dying, palliative care and euthanasia all too easily get bogged down by formal procedures, techniques and methods if not anchored in a global view on the human and on the responsibility that lies, or rather should lie, at the foundation of every concrete approach. Hence, in this essay we would like to develop a general, foundational view on responsible care for the suffering and the dying other. Our guide in all this will be Emmanuel Levinas (1905-1995). His concept of responsibility-through-and-for-the-other seems to us to be particularly suited to provide a philosophical basis for the interpretation of assistance for the dying and palliative care within the context of an ethics of caring. The radical ethical imperative shall thereby come to take a central position: "You shall not leave the other all alone in the face of the inevitable (death)" (*EI* 128).[1] In order to present the strength and the uniqueness of this view on responsibility, we start with the image of the human that lies at the foundation of the current, modern notion of self-determination. Only then will we be able to adequately bring into the picture the different dimensions of responsible care for the suffering and the dying. From the very outset, however, we would like to point out that our entire essay should be read along the lines of Levinas as a reflection that precedes the 'applied' questions concerning the way in which one should deal with assistance for the dying and palliative care.

---

[1] References to the work of Levinas are made by the use of abbrevations. For the full references, see the reference list at the end of this chapter.

1. An Atomised, Contractual and De-Incarnated 'I'

In the debate on euthanasia autonomy and self-determination take on central positions, in the sense that humans themselves must be able to decide about the moment and the nature of their life's end in a terminal or hopeless situation of suffering without the interference of others. However indispensable the suffering and dying person's own contribution and decision may be, and that is not at issue here, the underlying image of the human does indeed demonstrate a serious one-sidedness and a number of shortcomings. We shall enumerate these as the starting point for a broader, or rather essentially different, approach.[2]

First of all, the human is seen as an atomised individual that develops an independent self by means of thinking, acting and dying consciously and freely. In line with Descartes this autonomous self has immediate — or at least potentially immediate — access to its own desires and motives and, on the basis of self-determination, is capable of standing for oneself and coming to sound options and modes of behaviour. It is no coincidence that the famous 'principle of personal autonomy' forms the foundation of this image of the human and, consequently, is the condition of all living and acting worthy of the name human. This principle of personal autonomy, moreover, is conceived of as a right: autonomous individuals have the right to decide for themselves about their lives and the course of their lives, and thus also about the end of their lives. This principle of personal autonomy can only be delimited by the autonomy of others and by the damage that autonomous individuals are able to inflict on each other by means of their right to and exercise of their self-determination. The well-known principle of 'do-no-harm' is, in other words, fully understood and qualified based on the principle of personal autonomy.

As a result, the relationships between autonomous individuals rest on deliberation and agreement. This means that the relational network is secondary in reference to autonomous individuals. The intersubjective and social relationships are, in other words, preceded by atomised individuals — or 'monads', to use a term by Leibniz — who then in a second step involve themselves with each other on the

---

[2] R. DIPROSE, *The Bodies of Women: Ethics, Embodiment and Sexual Difference*, London — New York, Routledge, 1994, pp. 2-5.

basis of consciously discovered, formulated and cherished 'self-interests'. The ethical principle that must govern these free contractual relationships, on the basis of the mutually well-understood self-interest of the individuals involved, is the well-known 'principle of justice'. Transactions and obligations should not introduce nor maintain any exploitation or oppression. Furthermore they must serve very well the interests of all those involved, who in principle count as equals in the sense that everyone is free as an autonomous individual and thus, on the basis of this shared independence, is likewise of equal dignity.

A third aspect that belongs in essence to the autonomistic image of humans is the de-incarnation of the individual. The autonomous individual, who is posited as the starting point, is not only independent and stands for oneself or isolated, it is also rid of the flesh. The human person is entirely thought of from one's inner core, namely one's conscious, thinking and willing 'self-ness', which, as an interiority present-in-itself, determines the content and the direction of value and being. The autonomistic image of humans is, in other words, a spiritualistic human image: the individual person stands at the centre of the world as 'lord and master' (Descartes) and appoints oneself as 'spiritual and ethical giver of meaning'. In this approach the body has not disappeared but is rather reduced to an 'object' of self-determination and negotiation. We read the already famous work *On Liberty* (1859) by Stuart Mill: "over his own body the individual is sovereign". Autonomous individuals are the bosses of their own bodies, and thus also in their own bodies or 'in their own bellies', to put it according to an emancipation slogan. People are then also free to dispose of their own bodies according to their own discretion and enter into agreements and draw up contracts about their bodies with other autonomous individuals. In this manner we arrive at a subject-object relationship that is drawn to its extreme conclusion whereby the conscious, thinking and willing 'I' not only stands over and above its own body but also above all else that is bodily and material, and thus also above nature and the entire cosmos.[3] This actively meaning-giving mastery is only limited by two restrictions that have to do with rationality and the principle of do-no-harm.

---

[3] As an aside we can ask ourselves whether the problem of ecology, with which we wrestle today, does not ensue from this functionalistic and instrumentalist relationship of dominance of the subject towards nature.

What is not reasonable or is useless, certainly when it involves pain, should not be caused on other living, non-human beings. But above all, no (useless) damage should be caused on other humans, certainly not without their 'informed consent'.

This brief analysis makes it clear that we are in need of another image of the human. Well then, the ethics of care addresses this issue by means of speaking about 'relational autonomy'. In this, the emphasis is laid on the principle of 'discuss-together-and-decide' and not on 'decide-for-and-by-oneself'. In this manner autonomy as active self-determination is not denied, but on the contrary it is embedded within the relational network of the ones involved. In this manner, one also endeavours to do justice to the multi-dimensionality of every human person.

It is our conviction that the ethical thinking of Levinas can offer a particular contribution to the deepening of this relational anchoring and foundation of human autonomy. For that purpose, the starting point is our care and responsibility for the sick and dying other, with whom we stand in a relationship *face-à-face*. Let us follow Levinas in his explicit formulation of our responsibility for the vulnerable, *i.e.* suffering and dying other. We must remark immediately that in general, for Levinas, there exists no transcendental and neutrally elevated standpoint from which one would be able to survey everything and everyone. There is always the perspective of the 'I' and the other, and my relationship to the other, to be characterised as 'through-and-for-the-other'. In so doing both the relational as well as the bodily character of human existence receive special attention. We are beings-in-relationship, we are linked to each other. And note well, this connectedness precedes our active relationships and obligations. We are all involved with each other because an other precedes us and is already involved with us. Moreover, this relational involvedness, which precedes our consciousness and our free will, is not only a fact — a condition or mode of being — but also a gift, an ethical appeal that summons us to substantiate effectively and concretely that connectedness. It is precisely this ethical mission that comprises the core of our responsibility to be near and care for the suffering and the dying.

2. The Other Comes Towards Us as a Vulnerable Face

According to Levinas the ethical relationship with the other begins not with my initiative or my free choice but in the appearance of the other, or in the face of the other, just as he describes it. If we go in search of what Levinas means by the term 'face,' we must immediately heed a great, but obvious misunderstanding. When we hear the word 'face,' we spontaneously associate it with 'countenance,' that is to say with the physiognomy, facial expression and, by extension, character, social status and situation, past and 'context' from which the other person becomes visible and describable for us. The face of the other thus seems to coincide perfectly with what his or her appearance and behaviour offers to 'seeing' and 'representing.' By taking what is literally an 'option' regarding the other person, we suppose ourselves able to 'define' him or her, whereupon we then also delimit our reactions and behaviour. Likewise, in all sorts of forms of counseling (medical, psychological, therapeutic), we begin from a 'diagnosis,' from a methodically and technically professionalized 'observation' through which, based on our foreknowledge of symptoms -the images of sickness -we can propose a diagnosis with an eye to prognosis and treatment.

What Levinas really means by the 'face of the other' is not his or her physical countenance or appearance, but precisely the noteworthy fact that the other — not only in fact, but in principle — does not coincide with his or her appearance, image, photograph, representation or evocation. 'The other is invisible' (*TI* 6). According to Levinas, we therefore can not properly speak of a 'phenomenology' of the face since phenomenology describes what appears. The face is nonetheless what in the countenance of the other escapes our gaze when turned toward us. The other is 'otherwise,' irreducible to his appearing, and thus reveals himself precisely as face. To be sure, the other is indeed visible. Obviously, he appears and so calls up all sorts of impressions, images and ideas by which he can be described. And naturally, we can come to know a great deal about him or her on the basis of what he or she gives us 'to see.' But the other is more than a photograph, or rather he is not only factually more — not only more in the sense where there is always more for me to discover — but he can never be adequately reproduced or summarized by one or another image. The other is essentially, and not merely factually or provisionally, a movement of retreat and overflowing. I can never bind or identify the other with his or her plastic form (*EI* 90-91). Paradoxically, the other's appearing is executed as a withdrawal, or literally, as *retraite* or *anachorese*. The epiphany of the other is always also a breaking-through and a throwing into confusion of that very epiphany, and as such the other always remains 'enigmatic,' intruding on me as the 'irreducible,' 'separate and distinct,' 'strange,' in short as 'the other' (*AS* 81). The other is insurmountably otherwise because he or she escapes once for all every effort at representation and diagnosis. The epiphany of the face makes all curiosity ridiculous (*TI* 46).

Still, for Levinas it is precisely in this insurmountable irreducibility of alterity that the vulnerability of the face is (*TI* 275), and in this also the lighting up of its ethical significance. As 'countenance,' the other is vulnerable, and can very easily be reduced to his or her appearing, social position, 'accomplishments,' and image of health or illness. In its appearance the other can easily be 'grasped' and 'gripped'. We shall see further how the ethical significance of the face is precisely contained in this vulnerability.

3. When Suffering Affects the Other

The vulnerability of the face comes to the fore in a special, disconcerting manner in the suffering of the other. Precisely in order to estimate its seriousness and its scope, we first reflect on the experience of suffering itself before we enter into the ethical appeal that comes to us from the vulnerable face.

3.1. *Suffering as a filthy fact*

First of all, we would like to bring out the features of the 'fatality' of suffering. If we are confronted with the suffering that happens to the other we are confronted with something that is more serious than the other's experiences of failure and shortcoming towards their own attempt-at-being. For that purpose we compare it with the damage to the attempt-at-being (existential design, self-unfolding) by means of *failure*. After all, this still has something to do with me: it has its origins in myself, meaning to say in my incapacity, laziness or lack of courage, over-estimating myself or overconfidence, carelessness or mistaken calculations, a lack of sense of responsibility or even bad will. There is, in short, the experience of falling short with regard to one's own 'task-at-being'. As an attempt at self-preservation and self-unfolding I cannot indeed forget that gaps, imperfections and deficiencies are possible in my exercise-of-being. The cases of short-comings, of inferiority with regard to my task as 'auto-nomous', to which I appear incapable of giving an answer as to what is expected of me, form a daily, painful experience. In my being-active I cannot forget that I run the risk precisely through this activity of alienating myself. In that sense, I am only active on account of free will and not of omnipotence (*DVI* 79).

And yet this 'disquiet' is to a certain degree less serious than the fatality of fate, which affects me unforeseen and 'beyond my initiative' in all its satanic externality. In a much more acute manner than in personal failures, I am confronted here with my own impotence and defencelessness. Against my inner deficiency I can recover by means of adjustment and better tactics. I can become 'sober' and only strive for that which is 'attainable', thereby patiently postponing what is not possible today in order to accomplish it indeed by tomorrow. This patient postponement, however, remains very relative since ultimately speaking what I should be doing is 'to give it my all, my best shot' in the sense that I should be realising as much as possible my capacities-of-being and relinquishing as little as possible only what is strictly necessary. After all, when I am impatient, when I do not compromise and do not weaken my unbridled claims-to-being, I risk, in the final analysis, achieving nothing: "a bird in the hand is worth two in the bush!" Precisely on the basis of my inner urge-of-being I am driven time and again to surpass myself and my actual achievements for the better and the more adequate. The fact that I remain below par with my goal of self-unfolding remains challenging me to begin all over, to correct my failures, to try out new possibilities by trial and error which would have less chances of failure. This never-ending movement of self-surpassing is precisely that which is characteristic of my disquieted but not yet fundamentally shocked and questioned attempt-at-being: by means of the inadequacy and the failure I necessarily become, as the striving for self-unfolding, a project of deliberation and consideration, reflection and planning, anticipation and organisation. After all, everything is permitted except the 'im-possible'. In line with my economic, self-interested dynamics-of-being I shall set myself to think and to 'calculate' in order to figure out how I can recover from all the failures and defeats, and especially how I can avoid or evade them in the future, or prepare myself fully well for them. It is apparent from all this how failure ultimately still strengthens my 'identity'. Failure becomes the starting point for converting the initial energy of my attempt-at-being and intensifying it for resistance, efficaciousness, willpower, resolve, determination, in short for courage and unambiguous self-affirmation (*DEHH* 175).

Over and against the fatality of fate, which happens to me unannounced, however, I stand much more powerless. I become, as it were, more brutal than with personal failure, the weapons torn from my hands, so that the accompanying feeling of passivity and the 'blind rage' that ensues from it are more acute and harrowing. I would like to do something about it, but I realise that I cannot do anything about it. Against my will I must resign myself to the fact that I am not equal to the task. Fate catches me totally unawares that I have little or no resistance against it.

3.2. *To be affected in what one is: physical suffering*

In this regard, physical suffering, meaning the suffering that afflicts the other in their bodily being itself, is much worse than the economic suffering that befalls them. Physical suffering is clearly a way of being afflicted in oneself, which in no way whatsoever is still non-committal or leaves humans indifferent.[4] This is in contrast to economic suffering from which I can still rise above through one or the other form of asceticism. It is much more difficult, if not practically impossible, to distance oneself as such especially from serious physical suffering — *and* psychological suffering that encroaches upon the body — so that one is not (or almost no longer) affected. It is in the nature of this kind of suffering itself. Not only is it more radical than the suffering of the failure of one's own attempt-at-being because it escapes my capacity and initiative and thus affects me in my 'being'; it is also more radical than economic suffering: since I am only affected here as to what I have, I myself still remain out of reach and 'in-tact' so that after a needed breather I can still begin again and

---

[4] With this, we are not saying that we ignore the seriousness of psychological and psychosomatic suffering, which indeed can be just as serious and even more severe than physical suffering. The focus, however, is not so much on the comparison between physical and psychological suffering but rather the comparison with economic suffering. Since we are dealing with physical suffering, we actually link up psychological and psychosomatic suffering insofar as it is about suffering that affects human in their 'being' after they are affected in their 'having'. See *EN* 109.

'work myself up' once more into a certain 'affluence'. In the suffering that marks me in my flesh and in my being, however, my subjective possibilities and strengths themselves are affected so that an even more 'fatal' sense of passivity arises than in economic suffering (*TA* 55).

Now it is such that for some dark reason physical suffering, and *mutatis mutandis* psychological suffering as well, is often considered to be less important and superficial in comparison with the so-called 'higher', moral or spiritual suffering. However, it is precisely in physical and psychosomatic suffering that the 'being delivered and chained to one's own being' manifests itself unambiguously. In moral or spiritual suffering one can still preserve a certain attitude of 'dignity' by means of which one to a certain extent is already liberated. In physical and psychosomatic suffering I cannot possibly 'raise' myself above myself: I am pinned with my back to the wall of my own being. The whole acuteness of bodily and/or psychological suffering consists in having no single solution: I end up in the impossibility of escaping, of protecting myself from myself. I cannot command or force the physical or psychosomatic pain to go away. In physical and affective misery one is, as it were, forced to identify oneself with one's own being: one is ineluctably and immediately loaded with one's own being. The fleshly-painful vehemence of suffering hinders the 'I' from momentarily withdrawing into the unconsciousness and solace of sleep. This precisely creates the seething feeling of despair, which, as it were, forms the interior of personal, bodily or psychosomatic suffering. Hence this is experienced as violence: I feel myself gripped and overwhelmed by the 'other'; I become, as it were, crushed in myself, paralysed and reduced to a thing (*TI* 138-139). Suffering makes people 'unrecognisable'; often the ill person is so disfigured and degenerated by the illness that it is impossible to bear, both for the person in question as well as for those around him or her. The suffering imposes itself as the unbearable.

3.3. *Suffering is, to a certain extent, worse than death*

In this sense, bodily and psychosomatic suffering perhaps implies a greater and harder test for humans than death. Notwithstanding all fear of death, it still remains distant and set in the future. However imminent and surprising death may be, in the sense that it can befall

me at any moment like a thief in the night, it still is 'not yet'. In its
threat it remains in the future: '*Ultima latet*' (Montaigne) — 'The ultimate remains hidden.' I do not know when it will come. Even when
the end is approaching, death does indeed come as a thief in the
night... In contrast to the moments of my life that stretch out
between my birth and my death, and which can be called to memory
or be anticipated, death remains hidden as the last 'mystery'. In this
sense it is essentially separate from us as a radical alterity. For the
subject, as a being to which everything befalls in accordance with
one's designs and plans, death is an 'event' in the strictest sense of
the word: an event that is utterly *a posteriori* and against which one
has no 'power' at all, not even the power of denial. The future of my
death is an event that really 'comes towards me': it comes to me and
overtakes me from elsewhere, unforeseen and ungraspable, so that
I have no 'recourse' against it (*TI* 209-210).

It is precisely this future dimension of death, also of ineluctably
approaching death, that enables us to say that death is, to a certain
extent, less serious than suffering. Either death is there, but then there
is no longer any suffering; or death is still not there, but then I can
still pretend that it is far off. In contrast to this, suffering is an experience that grips me now and pins me to the 'present' of my fleshly
self, without any respite (*TI* 139, 205, 215). And in this pinning death
announces itself as real: suffering provides us with the immediate
taste of death even though death still has to come. In suffering death
is not only future but also present. By means of suffering our flesh is
marked by the sting of death. By means of suffering our existence is
not only made a mortal, but also a fearful, existence because, as
future, death is already present, tangible and sensible in my suffering body. I am afraid of death because it threatens my design-of-
being and meaning and eventually also destroys them. And note
well, I anticipate this threat in fear itself: 'my death' is not derived,
on the basis of analogy, from the death of others but it becomes accessible in the fear of my own being. Death touches me existentially precisely as the fear for my own death, meaning as my own mortality
and thus as the damaging of my act-of-being (*EI* 128-129). Well then,
this threat and fear acquire their actuality, full weight and incarnated
density especially in physical suffering and, in extension, in psychosomatic suffering, too, precisely insofar as psychological-affective
suffering also expresses itself bodily. Bodily suffering, after all,
announces deterioration and ageing, which ends up in death. Death

is brought closer, inescapably and terrifyingly, especially as incurable disease. It is enough to look up the medical files of certain diseases that are located in malignant tumours and the stubborn, brutal and, at times, unbearable pain that they cause (*EN* 109).

It is apparent from all this how suffering is not about the mere externality of death. It is not about, in other words, the mere factual ascertaining of the mortality of humans in general as the premise or 'major' of a syllogism from which one then deduces 'my' mortality. On the contrary, it is about a mortality that is lived through, which manifests itself in suffering. Bodily suffering 'possesses' the person from within and, as it were, in the flesh with the fear for death. Fear and suffering are intimately interwoven with each other. The fear that occupies, or rather 'is obsessed by', suffering is no simple 'state of mind', no mere psychological disorder and no pure awareness of finality, which would accompany certain experiences or ensue from them. The fear in suffering is utterly fleshly. It is the sharp point of bodily suffering itself. It is no epiphenomenon, incidental circumstance or side-effect. Disease, the insidiously spreading malady in the living but at the same time ageing body, deterioration and the unavoidable 'decline': these are the modalities or modes of fear itself. Through them death is now already present, really and 'lively', in our flesh as an 'unforgettable' and ineluctable threat. Through physical suffering we can no longer dissemble death. Suffering is then simply the unmasking and the truth of our existence, namely the disclosure of our utter vulnerability: we are in no way whatsoever armed and insured against death. Our is existence is 'without guarantees', which precisely makes it so painful and miserable. Suffering is the gnawing and the damaging of human identity, with all the 'seriousness' and 'weight' of a necessary degeneration and 'corruption'. Suffering then means the contrary of dualism. In physical suffering the taste and smell of decay are not added to the spirituality of a tragic 'knowing', suspicion or 'foresight' of death, however desperate this may be. Desperation and fear take place as *'mal de la chair'*, as 'malady, illness, suffering of the flesh'. Bodily suffering is the very depth of the fear of doubt (*DVI* 196).

4. Suffering as the Root of Abandonment

Suffering is not only the source and bodily expression of fear but also of relational and social suffering. In its fleshly apparition of becoming ugly, deterioration, ageing and illness, suffering literally works 'repulsively'. It repulses the onlooker and isolates the suffering one inadvertently: we would rather have nothing to do with them, we would rather look the other way. Suffering is the root of abandonment, loneliness, yes even of humiliation and persecution. We find a strong illustration of this in the biblical book of Job. When he was 'inflicted [with] loathsome sores' 'from the sole of his foot to the crown of his head' (Job 2,7b), not only did his wife mock him (2,9) but he was also abandoned by his friends: "My companions are treacherous like a torrent-bed, like freshets that pass away, that run dark with ice, turbid with melting snow. In time of heat they disappear; when it is hot they vanish from their place" 6,15-17). His suffering brings him defamation and humiliation: "Those at ease have contempt for misfortune, but it is ready for those whose feet are unstable" (12,5); "they have gaped at me with their mouths; they have struck me insolently on the cheek; they mass themselves together against me" (16,10); "he has made me a byword of the peoples, and I am one before whom people spit" (17,6). His suffering makes him literally into an 'outcast' and one 'persecuted': "He has put my family far from me, and my acquaintances are wholly estranged from me. My relatives and my close friends have failed me; the guests in my house have forgotten me; my serving girls count me as a stranger; I have become an alien in their eyes. I call to my servant, he gives me no answer; I must myself plead with him. My breath is repulsive to my wife; I am loathsome to my own family. Even young children despise me; when I rise, they talk against me. All my intimate friends abhor me, and those who I loved have turned against me. My bones cling to my skin and to my flesh, and I have escaped by the skin of my teeth. Have pity on me, have pity on me, O you my friends, for the hand of God has touched me! Why do you, like God, pursue me, never satisfied with my flesh? (19,13-22). And he is also laughed at by youngsters, who mock him with songs and gossip about him: "But now they make sport of me, those who are younger than I, whose fathers I would have disdained to set with the dogs of my flock. What could I gain from the strength of their hands? All their vigour is gone. Through want and hard hunger they gnaw the dry and desolate ground, they pick mallow and the leaves of bushes, and to warm themselves the roots of broom. They are driven out from society, people shout after them as after a thief" (30,1-5) (*DVI* 96-97).

4.1. *The excessiveness of suffering*

All this leads Levinas to label suffering as the 'excessive' *par excellence*. The term 'excessive', however, should not be understood quantitatively, thus not in the sense of 'intensity' that goes beyond a certain degree or measure. Suffering is not 'disproportionate' because it can be so strong and tumultuous that it goes beyond the 'bearable', even though we most easily come to be aware of its excessiveness through its intensity. Evil is disproportion in essence. In other words, we need to understand the excessiveness of suffering qualitatively, namely as a breach with the 'normal' and 'normative', with what is obvious or what lies in line with one's expectations, as a violation of the 'order', the 'syn-thesis', the 'regulated', the 'fitting', in short as the frustration of all that agrees with the attempt-at-being and fits with the dynamics of the personal project-of-existence. Suffering is essentially and literally 'ex-cessive': it overflows the banks of healthy self-unfolding. It essentially stands counter to the power of self-determination.

It is precisely this qualitative excessiveness of suffering that makes up its 'evilness', so that it is also not coincidentally — along with death as its 'scandalous completion' — labelled as the *evil par excellence*. In contrast to Scholasticism, which considers evil as a 'privation of being' (*privatio entis*), here a different and also 'harder' definition of suffering is given. Suffering is not so much a lack but a radical violation and disruption of being. It is no inadequacy but disintegration, no limitation but an unmerciful contradiction, which throws everything upside down. An ethics of compassion which would overlook this would all too quickly be inclined to trivialise suffering and explain it away. Suffering imposes itself as the filthy scandal of a decomposing force that spares nothing. It is then no coincidence that the evilness of suffering has been characterised as '*dia*bolical', which is exactly the opposite of '*sym*bolical', meaning to say that which binds, brings to unity, order, synthesis and harmony.

That is also why Levinas calls suffering '*l'inassumable*': that which we attempt to appropriate to ourselves and take up as a part of our design-for-existence', but which escapes us time and again. Suffering repeatedly disarms us, even though we try time and again to grab these weapons back. But even that again fails. And it is this infernal downward spiral of failure that establishes the evilness of suffering. Ultimately it allows no synthesis or order, even though there seems to be temporarily some 'order' now and then. Suffering is a filthy alterity, an indigestible heterogeneity and disparity. Suffering is essentially the refusal itself of all synthesis, even though we are for the moment — or even for a longer period — lulled into sleep by recovery: "that which disturbs order *and* is the disturbance of order, at one and the same time" (*EN* 107). And this radical opposition is no formal or intellectual heteronomy but a contradiction as well as perception: the painfulness of pain, unbearable and unacceptable evil, that submerges us into passivity. It is, in other words, suffering as 'experience', not to be understood as act but as even 'despite ourselves'. The passivity of suffering that affects us is much more radically passive than the receptivity of our senses that still exhibit an active passivity, meaning to say an intentional receptiveness, which then takes place as perception. "In suffering sensibility is vulnerability, more passive than receptivity; it is a testing, more passive than experience. And hence it is precisely an evil. Suffering is a pure experiencing" (*EN* 108). And the pain of suffering the expression and the realisation itself thereof, including the intense pain that swallows up consciousness entirely and reduces it to (almost) nothing. In this hellish pain, the wild evilness of suffering shows itself" (*EN* 109).

5. The Temptation to Pass the Suffering and the Dying Other By

Well then, it is precisely this pain in the evilness of the suffering of the vulnerable and injured other that an appeal breaks through, an appeal directed to me for 'assistance', help and care. And this appeal manifests itself concretely in and through the sigh, the grimace, the cry, the fear in the eyes, the complaint and the wailing (*EN* 109). There is something remarkable, however, going on in this appeal. On the side of the one who 'hears' or notices the appeal, it is not accompanied by a spontaneous, obvious and natural surge of enthusiasm but rather by a radical reluctance and resistance, meaning the spontaneous inclination to reject it. In order to assess the ethical appeal adequately and realistically, we must first look into this resistance and reluctance.

When I am confronted by the suffering and dying of the other I must honestly admit that I would not have anything to do with it and that consequently I would rather not be involved in it. The suffering and dying of the other, after all, upsets my attempt-at-being, meaning to say my existential project and my self-unfolding. This runs parallel with the experience of the suffering that affects myself. Propelled by my attempt-at-being I would rather not be confronted with suffering, an injury or an accident. As a finite being I am mortal, but precisely through my finitude I become an attempt-at-being that would do anything in order to be affected as little as possible by suffering and death. That is my struggle for life: I would very much like to avoid suffering as much as possible. This is in line with what Sigmund Freud said regarding the principle of delight, which — in confrontation with reality — becomes a selfish, economic principle: 'as much delight as possible and as little unease as possible'. I myself am written up for death, but 'for the moment' — and that is each and every moment, until we can no longer put it off — I would rather not want to be confronted by it. I flee from death, I live in postponement (with the — to be sure, impossible — wish for its cancellation). My existence is all at once fear and trembling, from which I try to escape by means of putting off suffering and especially death by feverishly investing in all sorts of activity or pleasure. And the idea explained above of the radical future of death helps me, insofar as I can live and act, to do as if I still had an entire eternity before me.

The same aversion and resistance also counts with regard to the confrontation with the suffering and dying of the other. I would rather not be confronted by it. We should link this with what Levinas calls the "temptation to kill". As 'healthy' beings involved with ourselves, who strive for as much happiness as possible and as little sadness as possible for ourselves, we would rather not be confronted with the suffering that befalls someone else. The suffering of the other inconveniences and disorders us, puts us off balance, disturbs our schedule, breaks into the world of our feelings and disrupts our tranquillity, whereby we lose our equanimity. We no longer have everything under control. The weapons of our self-determination are seized from our hands. The suffering of the other is the concrete, harrowing heteronomy of the other, who breaks into our existence unasked and impertinently. Of ourselves, on the basis of our own insight and ability, we find no way out.

We would rather be rid of it: "let this cup pass from me". There is no spontaneous desire to have something to do with the suffering and dying other. Caring for the other is no natural, idyllic feeling of compassion, which simply wells up in our hearts. Such a desire rather has something masochistic than realistic about it. We would rather turn our gaze away, or would rather go around, avoiding the one suffering or dying (just as the priest and the Levite do in the gospel story of the Good Samaritan). The suffering and dying other is 'to be avoided'. And this is a 'natural' reflex. This reflex has nothing to do with one or the other perverse, diabolic or sadistic personality. It is linked 'normally' — obviously — to our healthy, involved-with-ourselves, attempt-at-being. After all, it hopes primarily for itself, namely to become as happy as possible, and thus precisely hopes not to be confronted with unforeseen events that would disrupt daily existence, of which the suffering and dying of the other are eminent expressions. In this regard, the suffering of the heteronomous other is not only unexpected but also utterly undesired and 'un-natural', literally a '*contre-sens*', an 'un-desirable'.

To try to escape from it is precisely the 'temptation to kill'. To kill can be understood here in different ways. To kill can consist in reducing the other to its countenance or appearance. On the basis of my perception — whether spontaneous or permeated by method — 'vision' in the literal sense of the word — I strive to grasp the other in an image and to keep him or her in my sights. And this perception takes place not out of 'contemplative' consideration which wishes only to respectfully 'mirror' the other or 'let him be seen,' but according to self-interested concerns. When I thus succeed in discovering or 'dis-closing' the other person, I can also know how I can interact with him, and how I can include him in the realization of my autonomy and right to freedom. Hence does the face appear as pre-eminently vulnerable, in so far as it can be reduced — based on its appearing and on the ground of my perception — precisely to its countenance. In its appearing, the face presents itself to me naked; it is, as it were, handed over defenceless before the 'shameless gaze' which observes and explores it. The nudity of the face is an 'uncomfortable' nudity — one which testifies to an essential destitution. The proof of this is in the fact that the other tries to camouflage his poverty by taking on airs, by posing or posturing, making and dressing himself up, grooming and preening. This makes it clear that the other is naked, and by its appearing the plainly 'voyeuristic' I is invited to violence. By its 'countenance,' its visibility, the face challenges me as self-interested effort of existing to imprison the other there, in what I see: or, to invoke a play of words, the other who is seen, '*is* seen.' (*AE* 113-115).

We can also 'kill' by means of reducing the other, in one way or another, to the function or instrument of our existence and our own identity, i.e. a means to fulfil our own needs: "reduction of the other to the same" (*TI* 6), as Levinas pithily puts it as the characterisation of every form of killing. Committing violence is always a form of trespass into the irreducible alterity of the other, whether it concerns a form of use, consumption or abuse, or rather oppression, tyranny or terror. All possible means can be taken into consideration in order to draw the other to me, to possess it, to blackmail it, to intimidate or bribe it, to grab it directly or indirectly and to manipulate it (*TI* 209, LC 268).

In its extreme form, to kill is the act of murder, namely the physical act whereby one takes away the life of someone. Levinas even speaks of the 'passion' of murder, insofar as it is driven by a well-determined intentionality, namely, to totally destroy the other. The 'denial' occurring in the 'consumption' and 'use' of others still remains partial. In the 'grasp' that I exert on them, I do indeed contest their independence but I still preserve their existence in reality so that they are and continue to be 'for me.' Murdering is radical: one does not dominate (appropriate, use and consume) the other, but clears them out of the way, or destroys them; the other is driven even from existing. To kill, then, renounces absolutely all 'com-prehension' of the other, for one no longer wishes to include the other in the 'same' — that is, in one's own project of existing — but, on the contrary, to exclude him, because he is 'too much' in the way of my struggle for identity. Murder manifests itself as the effort and realization of an inexorable struggle for omnipotence: the I plays not 'all *or* nothing' but 'all *and* nothing.' It promotes itself to 'all' so that the other must be reduced to 'nothing' or 'no one,' which is also to say to 'is-no-longer,' in not only the factual but also, and above all, the active sense of 'is' no-longer (*être* understood not formally as 'existence' but qualitatively as '*conatus essendi*,' thus as 'capacity.') (*TI* 172)

To kill can also consist in excluding the other. To kill, therefore, as 'carefully pass the other by': to pretend as if nothing is happening, to make believe there is nothing serious going on with the other. To kill is to forget, to totally disregard, a complete lack of attention. Usually we do not directly say 'no': you do not concern me, or your suffering and dying are none of my business. We have learned our manners, often disguised as a form of so-called civilisation and 'politeness': namely making a 'small detour', so that we can pretend we did not see the other. But turning away our eyes or looking the other way is already bad faith, for we cannot make believe we have not seen the other if we indeed did not see the other. To kill is, in one way or the other, to deny the other, to abandon it, to deal with it 'lightly' and 'fleetingly' by means of relativising, minimising, trivialising the seriousness of that which affects the other. To kill has many modalities, and it does not always show itself unveiled, but it is no less real and merciless. It is apparent from all this how our attempt-at-being, in its natural, spontaneous condition, is potentially indifferent and violent. Left to itself, our attempt-at-being makes very little trouble to despise, avoid or ignore the other.

6. Called to Care for the Suffering and Dying Other

But precisely in this temptation to 'kill' the other or to 'deliver it unto death' lies, according to Levinas, the ethical significance of the face. And we would now like to explore in depth this ethical significance, paying particular attention to our responsible care for the suffering and dying other.

6.1. *The vulnerable face of the suffering other utters: 'You shall not kill'*

At the moment in which I am attracted by the naked face of the other, by its mortal vulnerability, abandoning the other to its fate, I simultaneously realize that which can be actually must not. This is the core of the fundamental ethical experience beginning from the face. Levinas expresses this as a categorical imperative emanating from the face: 'Thou shalt not kill.' In my self-sufficient effort of existing, which on the ground of perception and representation aims to become the expression and realization of individual freedom, I am not merely limited from the outside but at my deepest — in the very principle of my freedom — shocked and placed in question (*EI* 129). Here we stumble upon the bottom limit of ethics, namely the minimal condition for humane, inter-human relationships. It will be made clear how this bottom boundary line does not yet fulfil what an ethical qualitative care for the suffering and dying other entails.

Thus, of course, it is through its countenance and its naked poverty that the face can be killed, missed out, excluded or despised. And the fact that this is not only a possibility but an everyday — or even banal — reality is abundantly clear from our newspaper and television reports of violence, homicide, war, hatred, indifference and merciless inflexibility. In this sense, the face as ethical appeal is not an ontological or natural 'necessity,' like an object which, when let go, must fall, according to the law of gravity. The 'must' which asserts itself in the face -and by which the face is precisely a face -is not the 'cannot be otherwise' of natural necessity, but to the contrary a 'can be otherwise' which, however, must not. The prohibition to kill does not make killing — exclusion, neglect or refusal of care — impossible, even when its 'authority' is maintained in bad conscience over evil committed (*NLT* 22-23). In this respect, the ethical 'must', or rather 'not being allowed', is absolutely opposed to 'compulsion' or 'inevitability.' The face of the suffering other as prohibition does not force compliance, but only appeals. The face presents itself to me as an 'authority,' but one which can not compel me to anything, but can only ask and appeal, an authority which requires only by beseeching. The authority that reaches me from the face as a prohibition against killing is an 'unarmed authority' (*AS* 69) which can call only upon my free, good will for help (*AS* 69). The term 'appeal' expresses both the unconditionally obliging character of a categorical imperative in the Kantian sense, and a call to human freedom as good will — meaning as a will that can override its own self-interest and stand essentially open for the other than itself, but that can also, again as free will, cast this appeal to the wind. The face of the suffering and mortal or dying other signifies for me the experience of violence as continuous enchantment and real possibility, and thus immediately the ethical 'shame' that I must not be the killer of the other (*EI* 91).

6.2. *Care for the other begins as shiver and 'holding-back'*

It is apparent from all this how the care for the other does not begin as the positive movement of great zeal but as an experience of shock: the possibility and at the same time the prohibition to abandon the suffering and dying other to its own fate. The ethical encounter, meaning to say the care for the other, does not happen as a commandment or a behavioural norm to do something concrete. On the contrary, it commences as a negative intervention, namely as a prohibition, that questions the straightforward movement of the attempt-at-being. In the first place, I do not have to do something concrete; on the contrary, I am allowed not to do something, namely simply pass over or despise the other, or to deliver it to its own death. In this regard, the prohibition that ensues from the other awakes in me the fundamental ethical feeling of the *scruple*. The Latin *scrupulus* literally means a pebble in the shoe whereby one cannot remain standing but is moved or induced to take the following step.

A scruple, therefore, is a disquiet that works its way obstructively, or a shame and discomfort: I become apprehensive about gripping and doing violence to, about neglecting, about violating or destroying ('killing') the other in his or her vulnerability by means of which the other is delivered unto me. We can then label this first ethical movement towards the suffering other as a seemingly negative movement of restraint: "le mouvement apparemment négatif de la retenue" *(NLT 96)*. Confronted with the vulnerability of the other, I am demanded to rein myself in and to withdraw, meaning to say not to do something or, concretely, not to commit violence against the other or not to treat it indifferently. The ethics towards the other begins as the paradox of 'restraint', curtailment or 'self-contraction' in the unabashedness and energy with which our being-for-ourselves rushes forward, without looking right or left, without seeing the 'corpses' it leaves aside. Or to put it in different terms, the ethical relationship towards the other begins as hesitation and shiver, as a shame over oneself, as a movement of withdrawal and self-questioning: 'Oh dear, what I am doing…? Am I perhaps too 'vehement', too self-assured and insouciant, and only concerned about my own happiness, future and meaning? Do I perhaps kill simply by being?' *(NLT 22-25, 94-96)*. We would perhaps rather run away from the suffering and dying other, but we should not do that. Naturally, we can let the other suffocate in its suffering and dying, and people do that often, certainly in a professional and skilful culture like ours that wants to keep everything neat and under control. The fundamental ethical choice consists, however, in not obscuring or pushing away the crisis that the other causes in us; in not undoing the unease that the face of the other arouses in us by means of all sorts of techniques and strategies; but on the contrary to withstand that crisis and unease as a choice not to abandon the other in its suffering and dying. We do not flee from the 'crisis of our own being' precisely because we are on our guard for 'the easiness of ease' whereby we try to skirt around the suffering and dying other or try to — in a sensible, non-brutal, indirect manner — avoid it.

6.3. *Responsibility as goodness and generous care for the other*

The apparently negative movement of reserve and placing oneself in question in the effort of existing, so to speak, makes room for the positive movement of attention, solicitude and responsibility for the other. This responsibility, which establishes the non-killing of the other and which begins as from the summons of the face — and, finally, which is therefore radically heteronomous — Levinas characterizes time and again throughout his writings as 'goodness.' It is a term very dear to him, and of which the highest realization consists, according to him, in existing close to the other in his or her extreme vulnerability, in assisting the other and in 'bearing' the other. Levinas calls it 'ethical motherhood' in the sense that one 'bears the other in oneself until the other is born' (*AE* 95).

The situation of need of the other not only makes me sober by being shocked and questioned as to my striving towards self-unfolding, but also arouses the longing to selflessly dedicate myself to the well-being of the other. Here, this is not about a minimally normative must, expressed in the prohibition 'You shall not kill', or 'You shall not leave the suffering other to his or her fate', but an internal transnormative must that flows forth from the irrepressible dynamism of goodness itself. Having said this, we do not mean a non-committal must, nor a recommendation or 'good advice', meaning to say a possible choice that one could possibly make, without there being any mention of an ethical appeal. It is indeed about an imperative, but then an imperative that goes farther than all reasonable demands of an ethics of common sense, of our natural inclinations and of utilitarian reciprocity and feasibility. And it is about an imperative that is not imposed by one or the other external law, but it is an imperative that is linked to the dynamism of the responsibility-through-and-for-the-other itself. Goodness, care for the other that is actively concurred and taken up does not limit itself to a negative reservedness that shies away from doing harm to the other by abandoning the other to its fate — its suffering and death. Rather it unfolds itself as a longing to go help the other and to assist the other with all one's own capacities and possibilities in a creative way. The answer to the need and suffering of the other can only be an incarnated and concrete answer. The only thing I possess in order to meet the other in its suffering is my ability and self-unfolding, my capacities and acquired skills, in short my unfolded attempt-at-being. I should not set aside, stifle, repress or deny my egocentric being and unfolding, but rather turn round, transform and make it available. Meeting the other who is in need with empty hands is a vain and sanctimonious gesture: real and 'fitting' assistance is one that the other deserves. The responsible care for the other must 'become flesh'. True spirituality does not take place amidst people as merely spiritual creatures, but precisely insofar as they are bodily and worldly creatures. The incarnation of the human being is the possibility of goodness as aid and assistance, to which the other as a human being has a right. In this regard, there can be no talk of responsibility for the other, and thus of ethics, without the body. It is only through the body that we are sensitive to the suffering of the other. And it is only through the body that we can transform this sensitivity into action, literally into 'handiwork' thanks to our 'hands' and all our strength and capabilities, our labour and possessions, our science and technique, our 'habitat' and 'furnished world'. Concretely, this means that I — technologically and medically — must do whatever is possible in order to ease the pain of the suffering other. Adequate control of pain is anything but non-committal; on the contrary it is an ethical duty that belongs to the core of the responsible care for the other: "medication is my primary ethical duty" (*EN* 109). Levinas then calls the medical a primordial, irreducible, anthropological and ethical category (*EN* 110). And this tangible and professional medical assistance must further be complemented by and framed within sufficient bodily treatment, relational and social, existential and spiritual assistance (just as palliative care attempts to do).

This careful goodness for the other discloses itself from the inside out, namely as an inner urgency — as an internal must or 'not being able to do otherwise', that is at the same time a command — towards a fully positive and joyful dynamism of creative involvement in the other. We *must* even more than we must according to the rules of the accepted ethics of 'common sense': a nearness that is never sufficiently near, just as an embrace that is never close enough (*AE* 103). We realize that we must go further than what is required of us by duty. Or to put it contradictorily: it is our duty to do more than our duty. Radical 'diakonia', vested with the humility of one who has no time to care for oneself, who does not expect gratitude, recognition or reward (not even the 'salvation of one's soul' in the afterlife) (*DEHH* 189-197, *HAH* 46).

This unconditional and pure goodness, that does not care for oneself, is furthermore characterized by the longing to excel even more in (helpful, non-monopolising) goodness. To the extent I take up my responsibility for the needy, suffering and mortal other, the longing grows within me — and the duty — to even more substantiate that goodness and to extend it. The involvement with the other becomes ever richer and more creative to the extent it develops itself: an overflowing and endlessness that precisely expresses and fulfils the extravagance of responsibility-by-and-for-the-other itself, and which never simply lets itself be inserted easily and smoothly into the usual ends of 'legal or prescriptive ethics', whereby every form of legalistic conformism becomes impossible. Grounded in and moved by the appeal that the flows forth from the suffering of the unique other, goodness deepens and develops itself into a 'learning' and 'art' that constantly refines and qualifies itself, borne as it were by an 'insatiable compassion', *i.e.* a fullness of dedication and commitment that in itself is not dedication and commitment enough. The longing deepens and feeds itself as it were with renewed hunger. We can also call this the 'un-selfishing' of my unselfishness, literally' dis-interest-edness' or 'dis-interest-ing' as dynamic, ongoing process. In principle, I will never again be able to say: 'this is enough now, I have nothing to do with it anymore'. In this sense, my freedom is also deprived of its final word, just as it had already been deprived of the first word on the basis of the external origin of the responsibility-by-and-for-the-other. This exceeding — which has more in common with a transgression — of the law or of strict normative ethics that determines what is not allowed and what is minimally humane, can indeed give cause for perversion. One can go too far in disinterested goodness, coupled with extreme forms of self-sacrifice, that one lands directly in self-destruction and moral patronizing of the other. This does not prevent, however, that an exceeding of the law lies in the caring responsibility itself in the sense that its actualizations cannot or should not be laid down by any prescription.[5] Strictly speaking the commandment of the love of neighbour does not pose any prospective limit; on the contrary, it opens up a perspective on boundarylessness and endlessness that time and again makes itself endless, even though in so doing it is and remains a source of irritation and rejection.

---

[5] The way in which Levinas has described this endlessness of the internally appealing, 'demanding' longing of goodness, especially in his second major work *Otherwise than being* (1981), namely as goodness, taking the other's place, expiation, nearness which is never near enough, displays a remarkable affinity with the way in which the Christian tradition unfolds the dynamism of agapè as the core of the love of neighbour. This affinity refers back, to be sure, to its Jewish tradition, where Jesus and Christianity originate from — without thereby erasing their mutual differences and tensions. And yet Levinas develops his ethics of the responsibility-by-and-for-the-other as goodness that makes itself endless not on the basis of Scripture verses and faith arguments, but in a strictly philosophical way which rightly shows the general human, and therefore thinkable and communicable, significance of this ethics.

7. Not Leaving the Other Alone in his or her Suffering and Dying

Now, for Levinas the highest form of this 'goodness-full-of-desire' consists in not leaving the other alone in his or her suffering and dying. We can hardly deny that the most eminent and at the same time most painful human misery is *mortality*, of which our being in need of help and especially physical suffering signifies a frightening anticipation. We have already sketched above how death in the body that suffers pain is not merely in the future but already announces itself now. In bodily pain the other already is now inevitably handed over to the final, unrelenting enemy, up to the merciless paroxysm of death in utter loneliness and destitution (AV 196).

This is why we can rightly state that the 'fear for the mortal and dying other' forms the foundation of mercy as responsibility-by-and-for-the-other. The one who 'passes-by', as in the narrative, is so moved by the suffering and the being-near-death of the other that he has to give an account of the ultimate violence under which the other, in his extreme vulnerability as a mortal human being, has suffered. 'To see' the suffering other lying there means to be demanded not to leave the other alone when he — precisely through suffering and pain — is confronted with the impending death, even though I am in no position to fight against this unmerciful enemy and I can but respond with the 'here I am' of a lingering and caring nearness, holding tight the hand of the other, lightening and making bearable the other's suffering and dying, without the other being capable of returning the favour. In the face of the death of the other the duty to offer the other hospitality and to meet the other with giving and serving hands (*AS* 76) becomes the duty of authentic goodness and love 'without covetousness and selfishness': an utmost non-indifference, which in no way whatsoever longs for any recompense for itself. Goodness, therefore, as a non-mutual, asymmetric goodness that in no way whatsoever poses the reward or recompense from the other as a condition for one's own goodness. 'To fear the other' without this fear originating from the 'fear of oneself': "*entrée dans l'inquié-tude-pour-la-mort-de-l'autre-homme*" (*DVI* 248). A caring for the suffering and dying other who even bears to be vain and in vain when faced with the relentlessness of death (*EI* 128). This is only possible by means of letting go of the heroism of self-concern and move on to a humble, generous care for the other whereby one resolutely opts to assist, literally to stand by, the other in their suffering and dying.

Rabbinic literature even goes so far as to call this caring goodness the criterion of 'true mercy', which consists of loving someone as if the someone were dead. This does not mean that someone must first be dead in order to be able to be loved, but rather that we must love *as if* the someone were dead'. This is utter asymmetry or non-reciprocity. Then we can no longer approach the other starting from the idea of proportionality, whereby one does something in order to get something back ('quid pro quo'). When someone is dead he or she can no longer return a favour, so much so that I can no longer show mercy towards that other just in order to fare well in one way or the other or to expect something in return. The truth regarding mercy is apparent only in its utter gratuity (*DVI* 29).

This leads us to formulate, along with Levinas, a new categorical imperative as the foundation, orientation and inspiration for a humane assistance for the dying and palliative care, namely the commandment — or the unconditional demand — that no human being should be allowed to die alone. According to Levinas, every society stands or falls with that, namely to see to it that no human being stands alone before death. In the face of the unique, singular, other person, I stand eye to eye with every other person. In other words, it is not only about the close, familiar other, the member of the family, friend or loved one who is dear to me and with whom I have a bond, who calls me by means of their vulnerability and suffering not to leave them alone in their suffering and dying. It is also, or even in the first place, about every other human being: no one should ever be allowed to die in loneliness. No one should be left to their fate in the face of death. In other words, the criterion *par excellence* of civilisation, namely of a civilisation of love — meaning to say a civilisation of highest non-indifference — consists in that no human being should have to go the path of dying alone, even though no one can still do anything for that other. We thereby also ask ourselves whether delivering up the other to the principle of self-determination as the sole and highest principle is not a way of abandoning the other in the face of death. As long as we are not able to demonstrate the unconditional presence — simply being-with-the-other in their suffering and dying — there can be no mention of a fully humane civilisation, notwithstanding all other 'means of civilisation" which are conceived of and introduced in all other possible levels of society. And note well, it is not only the recipient or object of the imperative formulated that is universal, in the sense that no human being should be allowed to be alone in their death, but also the subject of the imperative is universal, in the sense that everyone — including every provision, institution, home for the elderly and nursing home, care unit and clinic, in short the entire society — should see to it that no human being is left all alone in their suffering-towards-death. In order to realise effectively this imperative, this radical principle, choices will have to be made, methods and procedures laid out and regulations drawn up on the basis of solidarity, subsidiarity, shared and substitutional responsibility. The imperative formulated perhaps seems to be a utopia, but it can and must become a efficacious utopia that is able to break through existing practices and call to life new ones. No human being should be allowed to die alone!

Conclusion

As long as I am more occupied with my own death than with the death of the other, the civilisation of absolutised autonomy has the upper hand over the civilisation of responsible care for the other. The difference between the one civilisation and the other is expressed, according to Levinas, in the question: am I more concerned with my own mortality than with the risk of being the killer of the other? Does one's own 'being-unto-death' — as Heidegger puts it — take centre stage, meaning to say my own fearful concern for my own existence that is threatened by suffering and mortality, whereby all emphasis is laid on the heroism of authenticity? Or does the care for the other as in the biblical tradition take first place? As long as the fear of being the 'killer' of the other, meaning to say the fear of forgetting the other or abandoning the other to their fate, does not succeed in transcending the fear for one's own dying, then the humanism of the other is still a utopia. By means of the imperative, however, which we in this essay formulated based on the radical thinking on responsibility by Levinas, the humanism of the (suffering and dying) other becomes a utopia that keeps us on guard by sowing in us a constant unease — an unease, however, that at the same time sobers us up and lights up in our hearts and bodies the fire of an inextinguishable, joyful surrender (*DMT* 109). This is the true vocation and challenge of every humane assistance for the dying and palliative care.

References

DIPROSE, R., *The Bodies of Women: Ethics, Embodiment and Sexual Difference*, London — New York, Routledge, 1994.

LEVINAS, E., 'Liberté et commandement' in *Revue de métaphysique et de morale* 58(1953), pp. 264-272. (LC)

LEVINAS, E., *Totalité et infini. Essai sur l'extériorité*, La Haye, Nijhoff, 1961. (TI)

LEVINAS, E., *En découvrant l'existence avec Husserl et Heidegger*, Paris, Vrin, 1967. (DEHH)

LEVINAS, E., *Humanisme de l'autre homme*, Montpellier, Fata Morgana, 1972. (HAH)

LEVINAS, E., *Autrement qu'être ou au-delà de l'essence*, La Haye, Nijhoff, 1974. (AE)

LEVINAS, E., *Le temps et l'autre*, Montpellier, Fata Morgana, 2de ed. 1979. (TA)

LEVINAS, E., *L'au-delà du verset. Lectures et discours talmudiques*, Paris, Les Éditions de Minuit, 1982. (AV)

LEVINAS, E., *Ethique et infini*, Paris, Fayard, 1982. (EI)

LEVINAS, E., *De Dieu qui vient à l'idée*, Paris, Vrin, 1982. (DVI)

LEVINAS, E., *Autrement que savoir (interventions dans les discussions)*, Paris, Osiris, 1988. (AS)

LEVINAS, E., *Entre nous. Essais sur le penser-à-lautre*, Paris, Grasset, 1991. (EN)

LEVINAS, E., *Nouvelles lectures talmudiques*, Paris, Les Éditions de Minuit, 1996. (NLT)

CHURCHES IN THE LOW COUNTRIES ON EUTHANASIA BACKGROUND, ARGUMENTATION AND COMMENTARY

Jan Jans

It will hardly come as a surprise to anybody even only remotely familiar with the general thrust and orientation of 'Christian ethics' that the question of euthanasia has been and still is seen in general as a moral disvalue and/or an evil that should be resisted. The bottom line of this approach is the theological notion that human life is a gift of the Creator and therefore a good to be nurtured, promoted and protected. Euthanasia, and especially its depenalisation and legalisation to different degrees in the current legislations of the Netherlands and Belgium, is evaluated as contrary to this requirement of protectability. Both during the (public) debate on euthanasia and in reaction to various attempts to legislate on this matter, Christian churches in the Netherlands and Belgium have raised their voices and addressed the public at large, their own members and politicians in order to influence reflection and deliberation.

In this article, I will first describe the argumentative way in which the major Christian churches in the Netherlands and Belgium have dealt with what they considered to be challenge of the demand to legalise euthanasia in their respective countries. Given the important differences between the courses of events in both countries, the part on the interventions in the Netherlands will be considerably longer than the one on Belgium. No doubt, the most important reason for

This article is an extended and adapted version of J. JANS, 'Christian Churches and Euthanasia in the Low Countries: Background, Argumentation and Commentary' in *Ethical Perspectives* 9(2002)2-3, pp. 119-133; J. JANS, ''Sterbehilfe' in den Niederlanden und Belgien. Rechtslage, Kirchen und ethische Diskussion' in *Zeitschrift für Evangelische Ethik* 46(2002), pp. 283-300.

this difference is the fact that the public discussion on euthanasia, together with efforts to change the penal law prohibiting it, took shape in the Netherlands already from 1968 on.[1] Next to this, the fact that the major Christian churches in the Netherlands were not in agreement on the proper approach also contributes to a more differentiated picture. In the third part, I will present some comments and a moral-theological evaluation of the core of the argumentation forwarded by the Christian churches.

1. Christian Churches in the Netherlands and Euthanasia

From my personal experience in various international settings,[2] I have learned that especially Roman Catholics are somewhat amazed about the differences between the Roman Catholic Church in the Netherlands, and the positions taken by the Reformed and the Orthodox Reformed Churches during the period that led to the first change in the existing legislation implemented in 1993/94. Therefore, I will begin by outlining these different positions, followed by a joint presentation of the churches' criticism of the government bill of 1999.

1.1 *Position of the Roman Catholic Church until 1993/94*

In general, the position of the Roman Catholic Church in the Netherlands with regard to euthanasia can easily be summarised: 'Euthanasia? — No, never'.[3] Clearly, the Dutch bishops are fully in

---

[1] See the study of the American historian James Kennedy who argues that the unique position of the Netherlands with regard to euthanasia can be summarised under the header of 'negotiability'. J. KENNEDY, *Een weloverwogen dood. Euthanasie in Nederland* [A well-considered death. Euthanasia in the Netherlands], Amsterdam, Bert Bakker, 2002.

[2] Concretely my participation as invited expert in a working party of the South African Catholic Bishops' Conference in October 2000 held in Johannesburg (South Africa) and as a member of an interdisciplinary colloquium at the University of Opole (Poland) in April 2001. See P. MORCINIEC (ed.), *Eutanazja w diskusji — Euthanasie in der Diskussion*, Opole, Wydzial Teologiczny, 2001.

[3] I am using here material of former research, see J. JANS, 'Argumentatie van de Nederlandse R.-K. bisschoppen in hun standpunten omtrent euthanasiewetgeving. Analyse en commentaar [Argumentation of the Dutch Roman-Catholic bishops in their statements on euthanasia legislation. Analysis and commentary]' in F. DE LANGE & J. JANS (eds.), *De dood in het geding. Euthanasiewetgeving en de kerken* [Death in Dispute. Euthanasia legislation and the churches], Kampen, Kok, 2000, pp. 58-65.

line with the *Declaration on Euthanasia* issued in May 1980 by the Sacred Congregation for the Doctrine of the Faith[4] and explicitly meant to support local bishops in their own teaching and in their dealing with civil authorities. The further audience of this *Declaration* is threefold. First and foremost, the Congregation addresses "all those who place their faith and hope in Christ, who, through His life, death and resurrection, has given a new meaning to existence". Next, the Congregation also reaches "for those who profess other religions, [of which] many will agree with us that faith in God the Creator, Provider and Lord of life — if they share this belief — confers a lofty dignity upon every human person and guarantees respect for him or her". Finally, it is hoped that "this Declaration will meet with the approval of many people of good will, who, philosophical or ideological differences notwithstanding, have nevertheless a lively awareness of the rights of the human person" (*Declaration*, Introduction).

The concrete argumentation against (legislation on) euthanasia builds on two lines: on the one hand there is the value of human life "[it is] the basis of all goods, and the necessary source and condition of every human activity and of all society"; on the other hand, and even more fundamentally for believers, "life is a gift of God's love, which they are called upon to preserve and make fruitful". The normative conclusion that follows from the position that each and every person has to lead his or her life in accordance with God's plan is also explicitly of a theological nature: "Intentionally causing one's own death, or suicide, is therefore equally as wrong as murder; such an action on the part of a person is to be considered as a rejection of God's sovereignty and loving plan" (*Declaration*, Part I).

In their important Pastoral Letter *Suffering and Dying of the Sick*,[5] issued on 5 March 1985 and written in the context of the hearings by the official 'Royal Commission on Euthanasia', the Dutch bishops

---

[4] To be found at *http://www.vatican.va/roman_curia/congregations/cfaith/documents/rc_con_cfaith_doc_19800505_euthanasia_en.html.*

[5] See DUTCH CATHOLIC BISHOPS' CONFERENCE, *Euthanasia and Human Dignity. A Collection of Contributions by the Dutch Catholic Bishops' Conference to the Legislative Procedure 1983-2001*, Utrecht — Leuven, Peeters, 2002, pp. 21-55. This collection is meant to be a 'white paper' containing documents prepared in the framework of the Bishops' Conference and give evidence of the "counter movement against the tendency to legalise euthanasia" (p. 10).

are following this pattern of the *Declaration*. With this pastoral letter, the bishops aim at presenting their reflections on 'assistance of the dying' — a matter that in their opinion is rightly a topic of broad discussion but too often gets narrowed to the question of euthanasia — to all persons concerned in order to give them a helping hand. Furthermore, their hope is not just to reach Catholics, but also to provide some assistance to those who do not belong to the Catholic part of the population. In the fourth part of this letter — after sections on assistance to the dying, dying itself and euthanasia — under the heading *Ethical and theological reflections* (pp. 39-55), the bishops engage in a detailed normative position. To begin with, the bishops take notice of the fact that the answer of the Catholic Church "Life has been created by God and we are not lord and master over it" to the question whether a person is allowed to dispose of his or her own life, is difficult to understand for many. Next, their own point of view is introduced with the thesis: "It is our conviction that such interference [mortal injection] is not allowed, because men must not dispose so drastically and finally of the life and death of another man".

The argumentation behind this thesis is both theological and anthropological. Theologically, the bishops argue that life is a gift created by God and that therefore between God and the human a relation of vocation and answer is established. From this, the normative conclusion follows: "No man must ever unilaterally break up this fundamental connection of every man with the living God, by taking his life or having it terminated, not even when he is dying. Because God is the creator and master of life. … Proceeding from the hand of God, we do not belong to ourselves". Anthropologically, the bishops argue on the basis of the dignity of the human person, being animated by a spirit and therefore self-conscious is both a someone that can be spoken to and is asking questions himself, essentially concerned and in need of others to grow to perfection and give meaning to life. From this, a — parallel — normative conclusion follows: "[A] man must not break this essential and deep connection with others by taking his own life or by having others terminate it, not even when he is dying. Because then he does not give his life back, but he ignores the deepest essence of his own self, that is: person in society. Man must not dispose so profoundly and drastically over his life".

Interestingly, this clear normative position is followed by a section on conscience: "What must be done, when a sick person in his dying process still decides personally to terminate his life or have it termi-nated? Here man's personal conscience is at issue". The bishops are affirmative on the dignity of conscience, also of an erring conscience, but they reject the notion that conscience is like an oracle that might put a claim on others to comply with a request for euthanasia. They recognise the ensuing tragedy for both the sick person and the doc-tor, but stress — also out of experience — that a refusal of euthana-sia if combined with the promise that dying will not unnecessarily be prolonged and pain will be alleviated to every possible degree is almost always an alternative course of action the dying person has peace with.

After the Dutch Parliament approved a change to the 'Law on Undertaking' in December 1993, by which not *de lege* but *de facto* well-defined cases of euthanasia became located outside the reach of legal prosecution, the Bishops' Conference reacted with a short but very critical *Declaration* dated 7 December 1993.[6] On the one hand, the bishops approve of the fact that euthanasia and assistance in sui-cide remain punishable: "This contributes to the preservation of an awareness that each life should be seen as a gift of God and that, as a result, human life cannot be treated lightly". On the other hand, they openly doubt if this punishability will be effective and they therefore repeat, explicitly referring to their pastoral responsibility, that "performing these acts — even when they are not punished — is ethically inadmissible". Furthermore, they note that the inviolabil-ity of human life has received too little weight in the public debate and they attribute this to the fact "that the Dutch Christians' have not been able to take a firm, common position". Next to their sad-ness that even some Christians assert that under some circumstances the active ending of life could be acceptable, the bishops also regret that even in their own Catholic milieu, the inviolability of human life is not defended with sufficient conviction because their statements on human suffering and death failed to have a strong echo. The *Declaration* closes with the appeal to unceasing help, love and patience of those surrounding the ill and especially persons in so-called hopeless situations "even to the end willed by God" and pleads for more intensive research in pain prevention.

---

[6] DUTCH CATHOLIC BISHOPS' CONFERENCE, 'Declaration of the Dutch Bishops' Con-ference on Euthanasia (7 December 1993)' in *Euthanasia and Human Dignity*, Utrecht — Leuven, Peeters, 2002, pp. 110-111.

1.2 *Positions of the Reformed Churches until 1993/94*

Before the government bill of 1999, the Reformed Churches in the Netherlands had not been involved in the matter of 'aid in dying' and a possible legislation in the same systematic way as the Roman Catholic Church. Partly, this can be explained by the plurality of the two main Protestant churches (in Dutch: *Hervormde Kerk* and *Gereformeerde Kerken*), but partly also by the different self-awareness with regard to the way these churches see their participation in a public ethical discussion, namely more as providing 'pastoral orientation' and much less as aiming at a normative discourse. The contrast with the clear rejection of the Catholic Church can be illustrated aptly with a quotation from 1985: "A request for euthanasia or aid in suicide should also within the community of Christ not beforehand be dismissed or be met with reproach".

According to Frits de Lange, there are two major texts that can be understood as a contribution to the ethical formation of opinion.[7] The first of these was the publication in 1972 of the Dutch Reformed Church entitled 'Euthanasia; Meaning and Limits of Medical Interventions'.[8] Written in a quite direct medical-professional style, its primary audience was medical doctors and pastors. In the context of the acceptance of the limitations of medical interventions, financial burdens are also put forward as an element of consideration. The ethical argumentation builds on the notions of autonomy, adulthood and responsibility; the theological core is the notion of the Kingdom of God by which both life and death are relativized. Or, in other words: there is no obligation to stick to life and in a situation of suffering one can lay down one's own life with confidence in the hands of God. The concrete normative conclusion is that both letting die and breaking off the process of dying can be "entirely responsible".

The second text was published in 1985 by the Orthodox Reformed Churches (although also supported by the Reformed Church)

---

[7] F. DE LANGE, 'Verschuivingen in het kerkelijk spreken — Verschuivingen in het euthanasiedebat [Changes in church teaching — changes in the euthanasia debate]' in F. DE LANGE & J. JANS (eds.), *De dood in het geding. Euthanasiewetgeving en de kerken* [Death in dispute. Euthanasia legislation and the churches], Kampen, Kok, 2000, pp. 46-57, note 4.

[8] *Euthanasie; zin en begrenzing van medisch handelen* [Euthanasia; the meaning and limits of medical acts]. Pastoral manual, accepted by the general synod of the Dutch Reformed Church, 's Gravenhage, 22 February 1972.

under the sober title "Euthanasia and Pastoral Care".[9] As the title announces, the style of this text was rather pastoral and its primary audience was the community of the faithful and patients, with the then contemporary political debate only being present in the background. To a certain extent, the argumentation is an ethical-theological mixture in which the notions of autonomy and self-determination are correlated with biblical 'stewardship' and the parable of the talents (Mt. 25: 14-30). Next to this stands the notion 'quality of life' in the light of which in some circumstances death can be preferred over life, supported by a reading of the sixth commandment from the point of view of Jesus' sayings about the Sabbath: norms are for people and their application should always take place in the concrete situation by means of the freedom of the children of God.

In the interpretation of De Lange, a more 'liberal' tendency was dominant in 1972. The text of 1985/1987, however, is on the one hand a continuation of this tendency — in correspondence with the societal situation — but on the other hand there is also a shift in the ethical and even more in the theological argumentation. The very wide perspective of 'the Kingdom of God' is left and replaced by a more narrow direct relation of faith with God, in which life is "a gift of God" that can however "break to pieces". Fundamentally, people of faith have their life in their own hands.

1.3 Positions with regard to the government bill of 1999

Through knowledge of these various positions of the Roman Catholic Church and the Reformed Churches, one can better understand the originality of the churches' reactions to the government bill in the fall of 1999. According to me, the government's self-congratulatory parlance of this bill being a 'key-stone' — by which on the one hand the proposed law with the ratification of the requirements of due care (Chapter II) and the function of the regional review committees for termination of life on request and assisted suicide (Chapter III) in fact confirmed the developments since 1994, but on the other hand also really amended the penal code (Chapter IV) — together with the very first words of the bill "Review procedures" (in Dutch: 'controle'), provoked something like a shock in the churches: termination of life on

---

[9] *Euthanasie en Pastoraat* [Euthanasia and pastoral care]. Appendix to *Kerkinformatie* nummer 159 (March 1985) & Vervolgrapport (January 1987).

request and assisted suicide seemed no longer to be a matter open to a discussion on principle but just something that is practically accepted and in need of proper regulation. Therefore, the reactions of the churches are not a repetition of their former positions, but an effort to deal with this new situation and exercise influence on the upcoming parliamentary debate. In comparison with former statements, there are some surprising shifts: the Catholic bishops limit themselves to a pure philosophical-ethical argumentation because they deem the matter to be of utmost importance for the whole of society; the Reformed Churches in a joint statement take their point of departure in the explicit profession that life is a gift of God and that therefore the tacit erosion of respect for life cannot be accepted.

The position of the Dutch bishops, dated 25 October 1999, is summarised by them under the catchword "Factual legislation of euthanasia" and is an empathic plea to "abandon this course".[10] The content of their criticism is as follows:

– the bill is a 'legalization' *de facto*: from 1985 on, the possibility for prosecution remained; now, however, through the power granted to the review committees the distance between euthanasia and the penal code becomes so great that the state is giving up the principle of the unconditional protectability of human life by creating a legal exemption from prosecution
– the bill is not a key-stone and certainly not a progress but an unacceptable 'break' by which the lawgiver — the protector of life of all members of society against any other member of society — comes in contradiction with himself
– the bill gives the impression that a request for euthanasia or assisted suicide somehow confers a right, but "it should never become possible to prosecute doctors for 'refusing to perform an acceptable medical action'"
– the damaging consequences of so-called living wills and the provision for minors to refuse treatment and/or ask for euthanasia even against the will of their parents[11]
– a lack of attention to the differences between euthanasia on the one hand and the decision not to lengthen life artificially and/or

---

[10] 'Reaction of the Dutch Roman Catholic Bishops' Conference' in *Euthanasia and Human Dignity*, Utrecht — Leuven, Peeters, 2002, pp. 139-143.

[11] This was also contested in Parliament and the only important change between the bill and the factual legislation approved on 10 April 2001.

pain treatment with the side-effect of a sooner death on the other hand
- especially not enough priority from the side of the government for dying with human dignity as is made possible by hospices and palliative care.

The position of the protestant churches, dated 3 November 1999, by way of a statement of the Board of the Together on the Way-Churches (a joint collaboration of the Dutch Reformed Church, the Orthodox Reformed Churches and the Lutheran Church) rests on the opinion that the proposed change in the law offers too little protection of human life because the borders of protectability are fading and can be summarised under the catchword 'A step too far'.[12] The content of its criticism is as follows:

- the present law should not be changed any further before a profound study has been made of the influence on the respect for life of the current regulations because it seems that this respect is silently fading
- euthanasia remains a transgression against an important value and should therefore continue to be a matter of the penal code; the tension for the doctor involved should not be solved by a review committee
- the risk of a shift towards the request for euthanasia, not out of actual suffering, but out of the expectation thereof, with the draft proposal in a way supporting this tendency, making it even more difficult for doctors to refuse the request or to propose alternatives
- the notions 'unbearable' and 'lasting/hopeless', are too subjective and may undermine the whole of the protection of human life (compared with the demand for 'late abortions' in case of a discovered malformation), also because of the influence of economic criteria and pressure against which the law has to offer protection
- a lack of attention to the protection of people with handicaps, chronic diseases and in a situation of increasing physical or mental impairment, whereas the greatness of any culture is the dedication to weak and broken life
- too much importance of a living will made years ago, and an overestimation of the capacity to decide for minors
- a lack of respect for the conscience of nurses and medical doctors and the risk of a split between those who want to maintain their

---

[12] 'Verklaring Samen op Weg-kerken [Statement of the Together on the Way-Churches],' to be found at *http://www.sowkerken.nl/documenten/euthanasie.html.*

oath to protect life strictly and others who will feel supported by a
broad law, possibly giving them an advantage in applying for a job
– the very important task to improve palliative care, instead of
enlarging the regulation of ending human life and thereby at least
attracting some suspicion that we are trying to escape from this
urgent need.

Although both these declarations elicited a remarkable echo in the public arena, their effective influence on the political debate and the resulting legislation was almost nil. In a kind of *ultima ratio*, the various Christian churches in the Netherlands, together with about fifty other societal
organisations, churches, patients' associations and other groups issued
a petition on 13 March 2001 — just a couple of weeks before the final
vote — and sent it to the members of Senate.[13] The content of the petition was an urgent appeal to reject the government bill, but to no avail.[14]

2. The Catholic Church in Belgium and Euthanasia

As I pointed out in the introduction, the differences between the situation in the Netherlands and Belgium explain to a large degree the
difference in the public involvement of their respective churches.
In this part, I will briefly elaborate on this and then proceed to a presentation of the position of the Catholic Church in Belgium with
regard to euthanasia.

2.1 *Background*

In Belgium, there have been isolated draft proposals on euthanasia
since 1984, but with the exception of the initiative of a 'National

---

[13] For the text of this petition, the list of its subscribers, a common press statement
and some further background information, see *http://www.sowkerken.nl/links/
euthanasielnk.html*. The concurrent initiative for an ongoing debate on the internet
(*http://www.euthanasiedebat.nl*) has not been continued.

[14] A somewhat different opinion was voiced a year later by the former bishop of
Rotterdam, Philippe Bär OSB, who stated in March 2002: "The acceptable evil is here
[in the Netherlands] well arranged". He stressed the difference between the moral
evil of euthanasia and circumstances in which such an intervention becomes understandable or even acceptable. See *http://www.trouw.nl/artikelactueel/1015827962430.
html*.

scientific reflection colloquium'[15] on the important questions of medical ethics in 1987 — an initiative without lasting societal repercussion — the real debate on medical decisions at the end of life and appropriate legislation only began in 1997.[16]

As far as I can see, both the fundamental and the factual drive behind the efforts towards legislation in the Netherlands and Belgium share the opinion that in certain medical situations a termination of life on explicit demand should be possible and that therefore a change in the penal code is advisable in order to grant legal security to medical doctors. Obviously, the 'publicity' in the Netherlands — including provoked 'trial-prosecutions' by and against medical doctors — stands in stark contrast to the lack of this in Belgium where during the last decades not a single real prosecution on the charge of euthanasia has taken place, although it is known both from research and from common sense that there are relevant similarities in practice.

Another important element is that the Christian churches in the Netherlands and especially many members of the Christian-democratic party CDA ('Christen Democratisch Appel'), which until 1994 was a leading part of the Dutch coalition governments, were not of one and the same opinion with regard to aid in dying and a legal regulation. Partly, this can explain the so-called public policy of 'tolerance',[17] by which it is recognised that the law as it stands is drawing borders that cannot always be maintained. Therefore, within this 'grey area' it seems worthwhile to allow for the development of a kind of dialectics between what medical doctors factually think that they should do when they are confronted with a 'conflict of duties' and legal jurisdiction. Eventually, a possible change of the law can be informed by and take advantage of such a dialectics. However,

---

[15] See W. DEMEESTER-DE MEYER (ed.), *Bio-ethica in de jaren '90. Nationaal wetenschappelijk denkcolloquium* [Bioethics in the 90s. National reflection scientific colloquium], Gent, Omega, 1987.

[16] See J. JANS, 'Euthanasiegesetzgebung in Belgien. Eine Übersicht über die politisch-ethische Debatte 1997-1999' in A. BONDOLFI & S. GROTEFELD (eds.), *Ethik und Gesetzgebung. Probleme — Lösungsversuche — Konzepte*, Stuttgart, Verlag W. Kohlhammer, 2000, pp. 175-187; B. BROECKAERT, 'Belgium: Towards a legal recognition of euthanasia' in *European Journal of Health Law* 8(2001), pp. 95-107. In this regard, the work of the Belgian Advisory Committee on Bioethics and its recommendation of 12 May 1997, have been important. See *http://www.health.fgov.be/bioeth/*.

[17] See B. GORDIJN, 'Euthanasie: strafbar und doch zugestanden? Die niederländische Duldungspolitik in Sachen Euthanasie' in *Ethik in der Medizin* 10 (1998), pp. 12-25.

many Christians were and are of the conviction that euthanasia, defined as "the active (deliberate) termination of a patient's life at his or her request, by a physician" and assistance in suicide are not under all circumstances a crime. Therefore, the question of legal security poses a real problem and the Christian-democrats did not as such reject legislative initiatives.[18]

The situation in Belgium looks different because the Christian-democrats of both the Dutchspeaking CVP ('Christelijke Volkspartij') and Frenchspeaking PSC ('Parti Social Chrétien'), who were always part of the government coalition, obstructed all discussion on a legal initiative until the middle of the nineties. Also, the official voice of the Christian churches is much more univocal than in the Netherlands because of the large majority of the Catholic Church. The praxis, however, is not so univocal, because of the awareness that good medical decisions at the end of life are not simple and that legal security could at least be improved. Furthermore, in the sporadic publicity through interviews or talk-shows, it is apparent that even well known Catholic medical doctors do consider a 'euthanasia-situation' plausible and that they would — in spite of the penal code — in some circumstances actually on request end the life of a patient or assist in suicide.

2.2 *The position of the Catholic Church*

Perhaps because of the (past) image of a tight connection between the Catholic Church and the Christian-democrats, the Belgian bishops have

---

[18] This also explains the at first sight somewhat odd fact that the 1993/94 change in Dutch legislation happened under the responsibility of a Christian-democrat Minister of Justice. See E.H.M. HIRSCH BALLIN, 'Leiden, Tod und die Rechtsordnung' in G. HÖVER, *Leiden. 27. Internationalen Fachkongress für Moraltheologie und Sozialethik*, Münster, LIT, 1997, pp. 263-276. "Die Tatsache, dass jemand Sterbehilfe wünscht, ist keine ausreichende Begründung für einen Eingriff in das Leben eines Menschen. Darin liegt die Bedeutung der Regelung zur Sterbehilfe, die in den Niederlanden zustandegebracht wurde. In Sachen Entscheidungen, die Leben und Tod betreffen, wird eine staatliche Überwachung vorgenommen. Diese Überwachung ist von äußerster Wichtigkeit: Sie ist das Herz der Regelung. Sie kann jedoch nur dann funktionieren, wenn die Norm des Lebensschutzes vorrangig bleibt. Es ist meine und meiner Geistesverwandten [des CDA's] entschiedene Überzeugung, dass es gut war, in Zusammenarbeit mit den Sozialdemokraten eine Regelung wie diese zustandegebracht zu haben: eine Regelung, die die Norm gänzlich aufrechterhält, die Berufung auf einen Notstand (im Sinne eines Ausnahmezustands) es aber offen lässt, Verantwortung zu übernehmen. Ich bin auch der Überzeugung, dass es Christdemokraten keineswegs schlecht zu Gesicht steht, an einer Regelung wie dieser mitzuarbeiten."

not felt it necessary to engage in political-ethical debates with the same high profile as their Dutch colleagues; the exception being the legislation on procured abortion approved in 1989. Next to the usually well-received and respected reflections and interventions of Cardinal Godfried Danneels, archbishop of Mechelen-Brussels, the Belgian bishops published two important statements during the nineties and of course reacted to the final approval of the law on euthanasia on 16 May 2002.

The first statement took the form of a pastoral letter and was issued in February 1994. Its central idea is very well summarized by the title: *To accompany people when the time of dying draws near.*[19] In light of this task and duty of accompanying — including palliative care — which really answers the questions surrounding the mystery of death, the Belgian bishops oppose the possibility of euthanasia because this amounts to reducing death to a problem to be solved. In an effort to reach all people and not just the members of their own faith community, they both discuss euthanasia out of mercy and next euthanasia as based on the freedom of each human person. In their rejection of these approaches, they first point out that euthanasia transgresses the old and ever valuable norm 'thou shalt not kill' and is therefore not a progress but a decline of civilisation. In addition, the bishops fear that the permission of euthanasia will bring about a deplorable shift in the vocation of medicine and that this would undermine the relation of trust between caregivers and patients and their families. In reply to the argument about human freedom and the situation in which the request is honestly forwarded by the patient, the bishops argue in both a practical and a fundamental way. Practically, they observe that dying people often suffer from depression and that the request for euthanasia is mainly to be read as a protest against the situation of suffering and anxiety; that the request most often disappears if the patient receives adequate medical, social and spiritual support; that living wills cannot be reliable; and that a duty to perform a requested euthanasia would fly in the face of the juridical and ethical tradition. Fundamentally, the Belgian bishops argue that even if somebody is really asking to die, this request should not be respected because no single person disposes over him/herself in such a radical way. Human beings are not isolated

---

[19] See BELGIAN BISHOPS, 'Mensen begeleiden als de tijd van sterven nadert [Accompanying people when the time of death approaches]', to be found at *http://www.kerknet.be/kerkvlaanderen/Nationaal/euth.htm*.

individuals, but always a being-for-another and therefore human autonomy becomes limited by mutual solidarity. Life is first received as a gift and also seriously ill people must be accompanied until the end. Furthermore, the bishops point out that it is possible — not just for Christians — to see the time of dying as the culmination of life, and that dying well in the form of exchange, friendship and mutual dedication should not be made impossible by allowing euthanasia but should be supported by those in responsibility in government, administration and health care facilities. In explicitly addressing their fellow Christians, the bishops remind us that God has not created life for death but for the future of fulfilment through resurrection. In the same context, they realise themselves that situations of suffering can lead to feelings of despair and rebellion against God and neighbour. Here, the task of religious accompanying will be both to situate this in the whole of life and to refer to Jesus who accepted his suffering and death and who notwithstanding his feelings of being forsaken by God died oriented towards God.

The second — brief — statement was issued on 9 December 1999 as a reaction to a possible change in legislation.[20] Referring to their position of 1994, the Belgian bishops repeat their support for palliative care and their rejection of euthanasia, concluding: "It is never allowed to bend this aid into the final breaking up of the relationship with the sick by killing him or her". Quite remarkable is the end of this evocative declaration, where after a citation taken from the encyclical *Evangelium vitae*[21] the bishops write: "In the event of a legal regulation, we are thankful to all those who engage themselves to approximate as close a possible the age-old basic norm 'thou shalt not kill'. Likewise, we point out that a legal regulation never replaces the ethical norm". Probably, this can be read as a support in the search towards a political compromise, which, however, has not come into being.

---

[20] See *http://www.kerknet.be/nieuws/templates/index3_archive.html*. A similar declaration was issued on 3 July 2001 at the occasion of the upcoming debate in the Belgian Senate on the bill, see *http://www.kerknet.be/kerkvlaanderen/Nationaal/03_07_01.html*.

[21] JOHN PAUL II, *Evangelium vitae*, n° 90: "At the same time, certain that moral truth cannot fail to make its presence deeply felt in every conscience, the Church encourages political leaders, starting with those who are Christians, not to give in, but to make those choices which, taking into account what is realistically attainable, will lead to the re-establishment of a just order in the defence and promotion of the value of life."

On 16 May 2002 the Belgian Bishops again issued a short but ringing declaration: 'Palliative Care: Yes — Euthanasia: No'.[22] Their reproach against the law rests on the shift between the fundamental respect for human life towards an assessment of 'quality of life', which introduces a basic inequality and signals a contradiction in the history of our civilization. In their repeated disapproval of therapeutic obstinacy, the bishops at the same time voice their support for palliative care even if some pain therapy hastens the dying process. They conclude that the approval of the law does not release us from the duty and the right to stand up for one of the basic principles of our ethics and history: 'Thou shalt not kill'.

3. Commentary

In the final section of this article, I will present my comments in four parts. The first is a kind of general moral theological perspective, outlining the framework I developed during about the last decade in dealing with the im/morality of euthanasia. In the second part, I offer some elements for further reflection on topics that risk ending up in the margins. In the third part, I discuss the requirements of due care and ask about the relation between doctor and patient. Finally and by way of conclusion, I engage in a critical discussion with the central theological argumentative notion 'life is a gift of God'.

3.1 *An old and a new question*

Because medicine deals with human life and health, it is obviously also involved with the end of life and death. However, in all the cases in which we have the possibility to act in a healing way — and in the majority of those cases, this means to realize a kind of prolongation of life — the question arises about what remains to be done if healing is no longer possible and the actual dying process announces itself. In a descriptive way, dying can be defined as the final phase of life or as the transition from life to death. The moral question about suitable or good behaviour and actions during this final phase of life could take as its point of departure the general insight that since our

---

[22] See *http://www.kerknet.be/kerkvlaanderen/Nationaal/16_05_02.html.*

personal dignity is to live out of responsible freedom,[23] this kind of responsibility is also applicable to the end of life. Nevertheless, it seems that both intuitionally and practically we have some hesitation to make this step. The reason might be the awareness that with regard to the final phase of life, we enter into a kind of border area in which special caution is called for and it seems therefore advisable to temper our inclination for interventions and actions and tend towards a more passive approach.[24]

The traditional example for this intuition and a definite normative solution is the so-called Oath of Hippocrates, in which is stated: "I will neither give a deadly drug to anybody if asked for it, nor will I council to this effect". For many hundreds of years, this axiom has been authoritative for medical doctors. It was strongly supported and even turned into an absolute by the Christian interpretation, based on biblical texts such as "It is I who bring both death and life" (Deuteronomy 32:39),[25] that attributed the exclusive rights on life and death to God and stated: 'Thou shalt not kill!'. Note that the correct translation of the fifth of the Ten Commandments in both Exodus 20:13 and Deuteronomy 5:17 is: 'Thou shalt not murder'. This does not mean that people did not experience conflicts at the end of life, but clearly there was a broad and deontological supported praxis — with whatever nuances worked out in the Christian *ars moriendi*[26] — in which the possibility of bringing an end to the life of a dying person was excluded.

A change in the situation begins to occur with the progress of medicine from the sixteenth century onwards — thus the speculations of

---

[23] See SECOND VATICAN COUNCIL, *Dignitatis Humanae Personae*. Declaration on Religious Freedom, Rome, 7 December 1965, no. 1-2. For a brief elaboration of the background of this shift in Roman Catholic thinking, see J. JANS, 'Enjoying and Making Use of a Responsible Freedom. Background and Substantiation of Human Dignity in the Second Vatican Council' in *Societas Ethica Jahresbericht/Annual 2002: Sustaining Humanity Beyond Humanism*, Århus, Societas Ethica, 2003, pp. 101-112.

[24] See J. RÖMELT, 'Autonomie und Sterben. Reicht eine Ethik der Selbstbestimmung zur Humanisierung des Todes?' in *Zeitschrift für medizinische Ethik* 48(2002), pp. 3-14; U.H.J. KÖRTNER, 'Therapieverzicht am Lebensende? Ethische Fragen des medizinisch assistierten Sterbens' in *Ibid.*, pp. 15-28.

[25] Pope John Paul II uses exactly this biblical quotation in his encyclical *Evangelium vitae* as general title for sections 64-67 dealing with euthanasia. JOHN PAUL II, *Evangelium Vitae*, Encyclical Letter on the Value and Inviolability of Human Life, Rome, 25 March 1995.

[26] For a contemporary reinterpretation, see C. LEGET, *Ruimte om te sterven. Een weg voor zieken, naasten en zorgverleners* [Space to die. A path for patients, proxies and caregivers], Tielt, Lannoo, 2003.

Thomas More in his *Utopia* — but gets into what looks like a rapids with the almost exponential increase in diagnostical and therapeutical possibilities from the middle of the twentieth century. Even if it is not mistaken to talk about a kind of 'medicalisation' of day-to-day life, I am of the opinion that these changes have sharpened our awareness of the coherence between health and a good life. This awareness is aptly formulated in the expression 'the cathedrals of modernity' by which academic hospitals are designated where we turn for care and cure — and in many cases also find. However: what if this is not the case and we realise ourselves in the midst of 'high tech medicine' that our course of life nears the end? On the one hand, the fact of our death is unavoidable and has to be accepted; an acceptance which for Christians by virtue of their faith in resurrection also contains the promise that death is not the final end of 'life'.[27] But on the other hand: even if death is losing its sting, an increase of the tensions and fears — exactly in the context of the 'medicalisation' of death — can be observed with regard to the road towards this death. Therefore, the plea for a humane dying or 'death with dignity' is indeed appropriate.

But: do we really know what such humane dying, or 'death with dignity' is? Hardly, I'm afraid. The opposite, however, the infamous cases where a loved one dies in a horrible way and death is finally a deliverance for both the patient and her/his neighbours, those cases we unfortunately do know. Those are the cases in which our moral intuition that human life has to be protected whatever the circumstances comes under pressure. Those are the cases in which also medical doctors and nurses — trained and motivated to assist people in their struggle against illness, bodily defects and untimely death (H. Kuitert) — start to ask themselves if the right to a humane dying should not also leave the possibility open to act in a way that terminates life at the request of the patient. Those are the cases at which it sometimes happens that the dying process is broken off and death is intentionally caused. Those are also the cases which whenever they come to the surface and are put to the test — in the court of justice

---

[27] In a comment on the Belgian legislation with regard to euthanasia, broadcast by Flemish Radio 1 on 31 October 2002, representatives of the Belgian Orthodox Church gave as their opinion that two 'moments' should be left completely in the hands of God: birth and the second birth which is the transition from this life to eternal life. In their view, the alleviation of pain can be accepted but both vitalism and euthanasia have to be rejected for strict theological reasons: the first because is turns life into an idol, the second because it means to usurp the place of God.

and therefore in the public realm — lead to the insight in the
dilemma suffered and open the eyes for the tragedy gone through.
And finally those are the cases which raise the silent prayer that it
may not happen to us — not as patient and not as neighbour — and
in which we always only hesitantly accept that confronted with *force
majeure* the choice for the lesser evil can be justified. And although
there is no precise empirical material on numbers of occurrence,
those cases do exist and they do not allow for any neat way-out.

3.2 *Some further reflections*

Both the Dutch and the Belgian laws can for good reasons be criticized at many points. The reply of the Dutch government, and especially its then minister of health care, that the law was nothing but
the key-stone to a process already going on for some decades, is
barely an answer to such criticism because it is also directed against
such a development itself. However, what seems to be forgotten in a
lot of this criticism, and especially with the accusation of the so-called
'dike-break effect' or the 'slippery slope', is that the factual behaviour of Dutch and Belgian medical doctors is probably not an exception and that a *direct* relation between legislation and/or jurisdiction
can practically not be ascertained. The concern that I want to put on
the agenda is that in discussing the legal situation, we should not
lose sight of the real matter at hand: the confrontation of human persons with the end of life and the ever increasing difficult medical
decisions which are becoming for more and more dying people and
their dear ones inescapable. My conclusion from this is that we
should resist the temptation to solve, in one way or another, these
problems by legislation: ethics and medical-ethical deliberations and
their proportionality can be supported or hampered by legislation,
but they cannot be replaced by it.

Another topic that deserves further reflection is the discussion on
'alternatives'. In the current debate about adequate medical decisions and actions in the face of death, one can only welcome the
attention devoted to approaches presented as alternatives to
euthanasia. My point would be that in the vindication of palliative
care as a valuable course of action or the admission to a hospice as
an alternative to care at home or in a hospital, the recognition
shines through that indeed the end of life has become highly problematic. This is especially clear in the context of so-called palliative

sedation as an alternative to euthanasia, because it recognizes that the patient is indeed in a hopeless situation including unbearable suffering, which is countered by an induced coma until the 'natural death' of the patient. Of course, it is the least of my intentions to diminish in any way the remarkable devotion of family members, nurses or doctors who engage in these alternatives. As already stated, I would like to raise and sustain the question if the experience of medically desperate cases should not spark our reflection with regard to those medical interventions which are bringing patients into such a situation. Also here, the simple wisdom might apply that to prevent is better than not being able to treat. In the context of Christian moral theology,[28] a renewed reflection on the relation between the traditional 'ordinary' and 'extra-ordinary' means and/or a development of criteria for proportional acting at the approaching end of life could be very beneficial. If I am not mistaken, it is exactly this approach and its corollary pursuit for transparency in all decisions that is the goal of the ongoing deliberations of ethics committees in Catholic hospitals in both Belgium and the Netherlands.

Time and again, a buzzword that enters the reflection on medical decisions at the end of life is 'autonomy'. From the historical point of view, the emphasis on the autonomy of the patient since the sixties of the twentieth century can be explained as resistance against what was perceived as the paternalism of medical doctors and as the search for a better balance, for example through the requirement of informed consent. However, in the context of the public discussion in the Netherlands and the political debate in Belgium, it seems to me that the appeal to autonomy as the key

---

[28] For me personally, the fundamental reflections of Klaus Demmer are authoritative in this regard: 'Wie es für den Christen keine Flucht vor dem Tod gibt, so auch keine Flucht aus dem Leben' in K. DEMMER, *Leben in Menschenhand. Grundlagen des bioethischen Gesprächs*, Freiburg i.Ue., Herder, 1987, p. 145 and: "The Easter event provides a key of understanding and interpretation in the task of making sense of one's death and of its historical anticipations. If death is not to be the definitive human and moral catastrophe, but rather a passage into eternal life, then there can be no historical situation, which stands outside of this promise and its power to transform. For the Christian, death and life are, at their very roots, reconciled with one another. There is neither an escape from life nor an escape from death" in K. DEMMER, 'Theological Argument and Hermeneutics in Bioethics' in E.D. PELLEGRINO, J. LANGAN & J.C. HARVEY (eds.), *Catholic Perspectives on Medical Morals. Foundational Issues*, Dordrecht, Kluwer, 1989, pp. 108-109.

notion to clarify 'whose life is it anyway' should be characterized
with the neologism 'egonomy'. In its reaction against real or pre-
sumed medical heteronomy, this kind of so-called autonomy leads
to a conflict between patient and medical doctor: the patient really
sees him/herself as a customer with well defined demands and
wishes, and the doctor as a competent supplier with the duty to
deliver. Although I know from experience that some doctors
indeed do see themselves in such a role, a legal establishment of
such rights and duties is not welcomed at all and the most obvious reaction is in the form of the demand for compensation and
protection by a 'conscience clause'.[29] Interestingly, such a conscience clause is not provided in the Dutch law since the legislator
considers that the independence of the doctor and his/her means
of resistance against claims for euthanasia are safeguarded in a
sufficient way by the requirement of due care. The Belgian legislator, however, seems to lack this confidence and Article 14 explicitly points out that the request of the patient or a written living
will have no obligatory force and that therefore no doctor or any
other person can be compelled to perform or to collaborate in
euthanasia.

Implicit or explicit: I would suggest that the phenomenon of a conscience clause in any legislation is a good point of departure to question the ab/normality of such laws or its underlying train of thought.
The obligatory force of any legitimate law rests on the generality of
its obligation, and with the provision of exceptions based on convictions of conscience, the legislator itself concedes that not all is right.

In the Dutch legislation, the requirements of due care with regard
to euthanasia are the result of almost three decades of interaction
between doctors rendering account, their assessment by judges and
a lively discussion between doctors, lawyers and ethicists on the
behaviour of doctors and the way it was judged. From this history, it
strikes me that three of the elements which played a role in this
process and which I would like to designate as 'circumstances' have
not found any place in the agreed upon requirements.

---

[29] A direct example is article 10 of the South African draft bill from 1999 on medical decisions at the end of life: "10. The provisions of this Act shall not be interpreted
so as to oblige a medical practitioner to do anything that would be in conflict with
his or her conscience or with any ethical code to which he or she feels himself or herself bound".

In the first place, there was the juridical notion of *force majeure* — an emergency situation in which the doctor can get caught between the duty to follow the law and the duty to assist a suffering patient with all means available. The acceptability of euthanasia by a judge in the case of *force majeure* is at the same time the forceful reminder that the behaviour under scrutiny is not normal medical practice and therefore the indication of its exceptional status.[30] Secondly, it is remarkable that the situation of 'imminent death' plays no role any more. If in the eyes of many, the plausibility of euthanasia increased by it being in the first place the shortening of the process of dying, nothing of this remains in the official formulation "ending of life on request or assistance in suicide". To some extent, the Belgian legislator was at least aware of the problem, because Article 3, §3 contains additional requirements of due care for cases in which "the patient apparently will not die the other day". And thirdly: none of the legislation leaves room for the — awkward — category of 'mercy'. This is remarkable indeed because it is not just a vague assumption that in the factual assessment by the doctor of what constitutes "hopeless and unbearable suffering", mercy plays a role. Of course, it is one thing to be clear about who is having mercy with whom and the risk of abuse should not at all be minimized. But I think it would be a step to far to allege that the risk of ambiguity is of such an extent that mercy should not have any role to play in (medical) decisions at the end of life.

As always with 'circumstances', their moral importance is dependent on the concrete situation. However, 'it depends' is by no means to open the door for relativism — this would exactly constitute the denial of the seriousness of the situation — but it is the expression of the always also present real singularity by which we are challenged to assume responsibility.

3.3 *Requirements of due care and the doctor-patient relationship*

In both the Dutch and the Belgian regulations, we can differentiate between two sorts of requirements of due care. Although one often

---

[30] This idea is very well worked out in E.H.M. HIRSCH BALLIN, 'Leiden, Tod und die Rechtsordnung' in G. HÖVER, *Leiden. 27. Internationalen Fachkongress für Moraltheologie und Sozialethik*, Münster, LIT, 1997, note 18.

can hear the opinion that these criteria have only a 'procedural' character, I would like to suggest that such a pejorative judgment can be
nuanced by making the difference between real procedural requirements and others that aim at the human factor in the doctor-patient
relationship.

The first kind of criteria is for the direct ethical assessment of less
importance because they deal with the practical steps that the doctor
must take to document and report his actions and how the inspection
by the (regional) review committees takes place. However, the second kind that really constitute the foundation for the decision to perform euthanasia form the ethical core. Here one should ask what
space is opened up for humane interaction between patients and
their doctors and if the requirements themselves contain some onset
towards the always necessary formation of conscience. In the following, I concentrate on the requirements of due care as they are par-
adigmatically formulated in the Dutch Euthanasia Act (article 2)
and add a brief comment with regard to the Belgian Euthanasia Act
(section 3).

a. "[The physician] holds the conviction that the request by the
patient was voluntary and well-considered". This first requirement
immediately makes clear how the relation between doctor and
patient is structured: the request by the patient is the indispensable
requisite but not decisive from the point of view of the doctor
because it remains fully his/her task to estimate the quality of the
request. However, no criteria are mentioned for this 'conviction' of
the physician nor is it clear if 'well-considered' means that the
request has to be repeated or put down in writing.[31] One can add
to this the fact that also the recent investigation of the practice of
euthanasia shows that in 39% of cases the request leads to termination of life (37% in 1995/1996). In about 20%, the physician
refuses, mainly because s/he lacks the conviction that the requirements have been sufficiently fulfilled; in the majority of the remaining cases the patient died during the process of deliberation.[32]

---

[31] From the yearly reports of the regional review committees, it seems that these
do play a role in the assessment.

[32] See G. VAN DER WAL et al., *Medische besluitvorming aan het einde van het leven. De
praktijk en de toetsingsprocedure euthanasie* [Medical decisionmaking at the end of life.
Euthanasia practice and the review procedure], Utrecht, De Tijdstroom, 2003, pp. 52-
53, p. 183.

b. "[The physician] holds the conviction that the patient's suffering was lasting and unbearable". A better translation for 'lasting' might be 'without perspective' because the Dutch original text reads 'uitzichtloos', but as far as I can see, the meaning is without ambiguity: 'lasting' means that the patient is in a medical situation for which there is no further therapeutical treatment available (some would even suggest that to continue treatment would come close to therapeutic obstinacy). 'Unbearable' is an assessment made by the patient but it is again the physician who has to agree and hence be convinced.

c. "[The physician] has informed the patient about the situation he was in and about his prospects." This third requirement is really but the rightful formulation of informed consent. From the point of view of the doctor-patient relationship, it is the precondition for an adequate approach to the next requirement.

d. "[The physician] and the patient hold the conviction that there was no other reasonable solution for the situation he was in." In this requirement, the dialogical relation between physician and patient is really centre stage and this can only be greeted. However, next to the lack of criteria for the requested conviction of both, one has to ask about the meaning of 'reasonable'. Does this mean that doctor and patient are confronted with a factual lack of alternatives, such as palliative care or the admission to a hospice? Or, does it mean that when a patient refrains from considering alternatives, this also counts as 'reasonable'? Opinions on this are rather divided and the vague formulation of the law allows for a wide margin on the side of the doctor without however providing elements of orientation.

e. "[The physician] has consulted at least one other, independent physician who has seen the patient and has given his written opinion on the requirements of due care, referred to in parts a — d". This criterion can be seen as a counterpart for the risk that the required 'convictions' could be overly subjective. However, what the law leaves open, is if the consultant physician has to agree with the attending doctor on his/her convictions with regard to the parts a — d. From the reports of the regional review committees, it becomes clear that if the consulting physician disagrees with the conviction about the patient's 'lasting and unbearable suffering', the attending doctor will ask for a second opinion.

The efforts to improve on the quality of this consultation lead to the establishment of SCEN[33] — Support and Consultation on Euthanasia in the Netherlands — a programme by the Royal Dutch Society for Medicine to train physicians for this kind of consultations. From the recent investigation, one can learn that the involvement of a SCEN physician raises the readiness of the doctor to report to the review committee.[34] However, it remains highly controversial if this kind of professional consultation results in a decrease of the actual number of euthanasia, because patient and attending doctor are faced with a 'reasonable solution' they themselves were not aware of.[35]

f.   "[The physician] has terminated a life or assisted in a suicide with due care". The formulation of this final requirement is also very open, but by this explicit inclusion in the legislation, it signals that 'due care' in this case contains the effectiveness of the means used.[36] Practically, it requires the doctor to be present at the factual act of euthanasia or the assisted suicide.

I hope that this brief commentary already shows that these requirements of due care contain quite some 'air'. However, they are not a straitjacket but allow for the space necessary in any doctor-patient relation. Building on this, an ethical dealing with the legislation could use this space to elaborate the intersubjectivity between patient and physician as the occasion for a formation of conscience without being 'sure' beforehand what the outcome will be. This kind of openness is to an important degree even more present in the Belgian legislation and in the reactions of Caritas Catholica and the university hospital of the Catholic University of Leuven.[37] The insistence to enlarge the circle of those consulted should not be seen as an effort to make sure that euthanasia is ruled out, but as an effort that real alternatives are indeed known and presented as real, including the whole range of

---

[33] See *http://www.scen.nl*.

[34] See G. VAN DER WAL et al., *Medische besluitvorming aan het einde van het leven. De praktijk en de toetsingsprocedure euthanasie* [Medical decisionmaking at the end of life. The practice and reviewprocedure for euthanasia], pp. 146-152, p. 200.

[35] See *Ibid.*, pp. 88-101, pp. 197-198.

[36] The Dutch Royal Society for Pharmacology (KNMP) has issued some guidelines but these are not accessible for non-members.

[37] For the position of Caritas Catholica, see the contribution of Chris Gastmans in this volume, pp. 205-225. The hospital issued a press statement on 21 May 2002.

'palliative sedation'.[38] Although it might sound strange to some, my own conclusion would be that the admonition of the Belgian bishops "that a legal regulation never replaces the ethical norm" is certainly not only not contradicted by these requirements of due care but that they can contribute to a truly ethical approach.

3.4 *Life is a gift of God*

On purpose, the conclusion of this article deals with the central theological theme that arises time and again in Christian positions regarding euthanasia, namely the thesis that life is a gift of God and its normative corollaries.

The specific Christian faith in God is literally the gospel — the good news — of God's philanthropy: God's association with and love of humankind.[39] This association of God with 'the cause of humankind' therefore transforms the whole area of the way we deal with one another in responsible freedom into a component of the content of this faith itself. The realm of the ethical and our engagement therefore cannot be seen as some kind of option or as something that can be left to the concern of others. This means: not just as citizens of a pluralist democratic state, but exactly as believers in a God whose glory is humankind alive, Christians and therefore also their churches cannot but move to the open forum of public debate and present their own point of view. However, and this is essential for me as a moral theologian, it is of utmost importance that Christians themselves reflect on the relation that surfaces between our broad, optimistic and inviting anthropology — this is why Catholics can address 'all people of good will' — and a normative image of God. On the one hand, and in line with the approach initiated by Vatican II's Pastoral Constitution on the Church in the Contemporary World *Gaudium et spes* (and worked out by post-conciliar moral theology) of the so-called theonomous autonomy, in which God's philanthropy is the transcendental foundation and *conditio sine qua non* of categorical human responsible freedom, God and humankind are

---

[38] See the contribution of Bert Broeckaert and Rien Janssens in this volume, pp. 35-69.

[39] See R. BURGGRAEVE, *Ethiek en passie. Over de radicaliteit van christelijk engagement* [Ethics and passion. On the radical nature of christian commitment], Tielt, Lannoo, 2000, pp. 17-50.

conceived of as *co-creator*. On the other hand, however, it is also possible that theological argumentations clash with ethical reflection and insight because this image of God leads to a conflict of liability or even a downright competition between humankind and God.[40] For, not a few Christians who take the ethical component of their faith with utmost seriousness have difficulty resisting the temptation of the so-called 'Christian advantage'. This is the temptation to introduce into the struggle with the grey area of (new) ethical quandaries a normative conception of faith that offers a seemingly clear answer but that in reality sells short the problem as an *ethical* dilemma by withdrawing it from the responsibility of human beings. Such a normative conception of faith no longer leads to (and sustains) a passion for the cause of ethics, but to a short circuit between ethics and faith.

In the concrete debate on the im/morality of euthanasia, this happens by filling out the fundamental anthropological notion that life is a *gift* of God by the theological normative statement that God as Creator and Lord of life is also its *Owner* who possesses the exclusive *rights* with regard to life — and death. From such a notion, both euthanasia and suicide appear utterly immoral because they are a direct infringement on these rights of God and God's dominion.[41] Often, the reaction to this type of argumentation is ethically exactly as arid by simply reversing the roles: not God but human beings themselves are the owners of life and therefore they can — for example in situations of (hopeless and unbearable) suffering — dispose of life. The confrontation between these positions is most clear in the temporal field: whereas the first approach holds that life should continue until "the end willed by God" or even defines euthanasia as "to take control of death and bring it about before its time",[42] the other approach claims that to dispose of one's own life and to die at the moment of one's own choice is the zenith of human moral maturity.

---

[40] See J. JANS, 'God or Man? Normative Theology in the Instruction 'Donum Vitae' in *Louvain Studies* 17(1992), pp. 48-64; ID., 'Het uur van de waarheid. Over consensus en dissensus in de moraaltheologie [The hour of truth. On consensus and dissensus in moral theology]' in H. BECK & K.-W. MERKS (eds.), *Over moed. De deugd van de grenservaring en grensoverschrijding* [On courage. The virtue of borderline experience and crossing boundaries], Budel, Damon, 2001, pp. 198-210.

[41] For an in-depth study of this, see W. WOLBERT, *Du sollst nicht töten. Systematische Überlegungen zum Tötungsverbot*, Freiburg i. Br., Herder, 2000.

[42] JOHN PAUL II, *Evangelium Vitae*, Encyclical Letter on the Value and Inviolability of Human Life, Rome, 25 March 1995, no. 64.

Replying to this kind of hierarchical antagonism, I would suggest that exactly the recognition and the thankfulness for life as a gift turns whatever discussion about who 'owns' life and who is therefore in possession of rights to dispose of life, into pointlessness. However, this very notion that life is a gift clarifies and sustains the responsibility of those who receive it. I will try to illustrate this thesis by an — as always only partially conclusive — analogy.

Each of us owns or possesses some objects: for example my digital watch and my wedding ring. What kind of responsibility do I have for these belongings? I bought the watch myself and as owner I can really dispose of it. Just suppose somebody would be fascinated by its radio-controlled adjustment, the double time indication, the memory functions, etc., well: I could give it away. The ring however (although I bought that too) is in the first place a gift: given to me by a special person at a special occasion and as such being the expression of special vows exchanged. Not just my wife would be astonished if I would tell her: "Well, you know, s/he thought it was such a beautiful ring that I gave it away". I also could swap the watch, for example for a nicer one, but to exchange the ring even for one that would be more beautiful really amounts to the proverbial wringing shoe. And to sell: no problem at all with regard to the watch, nearly unthinkable for the ring. However: *nearly* unthinkable, because the very special responsibility that really commits myself to it, could in the light of some circumstances require the exceptional measure of selling it, for example if it would be the only way to procure money to save my wife's life. An act like that is done out of emergency, as a lesser evil, but without losing all kind of responsibility for it — if only by a prevention of such circumstances or by the search for alternatives.

Life as a gift — for people of (Christian) faith even in thankfulness God's gift — is at the disposal of nobody. The responsibility for this gift, however, is really in our hands. Given the increasing need for ethical decisions at the end of life and in our striving for a 'good death', we would be wise to learn how to live with this responsibility.[43]

---

[43] For an attempt, see J. Jans, 'Tussen leven en dood. Contouren van een moraaltheologie van het sterven [Between life and death. Contours of a moral theology of dying]' in H. Beck & W. Weren (eds.), *Over leven. Leven en overleven in lagen* [On life. Living and surviving in layers], Budel, Damon, 2002, pp. 156-168.

References

BROECKAERT, B., 'Belgium: Towards a Legal Recognition of Euthanasia' in *European Journal of Health Law* 8(2001), pp. 95-107.

BURGGRAEVE, R., *Ethiek en passie. Over de radicaliteit van christelijk engagement* [Ethics and passion. On the radical nature of christian commitment], Tielt, Lannoo, 2000.

DE LANGE, F., 'Verschuivingen in het kerkelijk spreken — Verschuivingen in het euthanasiedebat [Changes in church teaching — changes in the euthanasia debate]' in F. DE LANGE & J. JANS (eds.), *De dood in het geding. Euthanasiewetgeving en de kerken* [Death in Dispute. Euthanasia legislation and the churches], Kampen, Kok, 2000, pp. 46-57.

DEMEESTER-DE MEYER, W. (ed.), *Bio-ethica in de jaren '90. Nationaal wetenschappelijk denkcolloquium* [Bioethics in the 90s. National reflection scientific colloquium], Gent, Omega, 1987.

DEMMER, K., *Leben in Menschenhand. Grundlagen des bioethischen Gesprächs*, Freiburg i.Ue., Herder, 1987.

DEMMER, K., 'Theological Argument and Hermeneutics in Bioethics' in E.D. PELLEGRINO, J. LANGAN & J.C. HARVEY (eds.), *Catholic Perspectives on Medical Morals. Foundational Issues*, Dordrecht, Kluwer, 1989, pp. 103-122.

DUTCH CATHOLIC BISHOPS' CONFERENCE, *Euthanasia and Human Dignity. A Collection of Contributions by the Dutch Catholic Bishops' Conference to the Legislative Procedure 1983-2001*, Utrecht — Leuven, Peeters, 2002.

GORDIJN, B., 'Euthanasie: strafbar und doch zugestanden? Die niederländische Duldungspolitik in Sachen Euthanasie' in *Ethik in der Medizin* 10(1998), pp. 12-25.

HIRSCH BALLIN, E.H.M., 'Leiden, Tod und die Rechtsordnung' in G. Höver, *Leiden. 27. Internationalen Fachkongress für Moraltheologie und Sozialethik*, Münster, LIT, 1997, pp. 263-276.

JANS, J., 'God or Man? Normative Theology in the Instruction 'Donum Vitae'' in *Louvain Studies* 17(1992), pp. 48-64.

JANS, J., 'Euthanasiegesetzgebung in Belgien. Eine Übersicht über die politisch-ethische Debatte 1997-1999' in A. BONDOLFI & S. GROTEFELD (eds.), *Ethik und Gesetzgebung. Probleme — Lösungsversuche — Konzepte*, Stuttgart, Verlag W. Kohlhammer, 2000, pp. 175-187.

JANS, J., 'Argumentatie van de Nederlandse R.-K. Bisschoppen in hun standpunten omtrent euthanasiewetgeving. Analyse en commentaar [Argumentation of the Dutch Roman-Catholic bishops in their statements on euthanasia legislation. Analysis and commentary]' in F. DE LANGE & J. JANS (eds.), *De dood in het geding. Euthanasiewetgeving en de kerken* [Euthanasia legislation and the churches], Kampen, Kok, 2000, pp. 58-65.

JANS, J., 'Het uur van de waarheid. Over consensus en dissensus in de moraaltheologie [The hour of truth. On consensus and dissensus in moral theology]' in H. BECK & K.-W. MERKS (eds.), *Over moed. De deugd van de grenservaring en grensoverschrijding* [On courage. The virtue of borderline experience and crossing boundaries], Budel, Damon, 2001, pp. 198-210.

JANS, J., 'Christian Churches and Euthanasia in the Low Countries: Background, Argumentation and Commentary' in *Ethical Perspectives* 9(2002)2-3, pp. 119-133.

JANS, J., "Sterbehilfe' in den Niederlanden und Belgien. Rechtslage, Kirchen und ethische Diskussion' in *Zeitschrift für Evangelische Ethik* 46(2002), pp. 283-300.

JANS, J., 'Tussen leven en dood. Contouren van een moraaltheologie van het sterven [Between life and death. Contoures of a moral theology of dying]' in H. BECK & W. WEREN (eds.), *Over leven. Leven en overleven in lagen* [On life. Living and surviving in layers], Budel, Damon, 2002, pp. 156-168.

JANS, J., 'Enjoying and Making Use of a Responsible Freedom. Background and Substantiation of Human Dignity in the Second Vatican Council' in *Societas Ethica Jahresbericht/Annual 2002: Sustaining Humanity Beyond Humanism*, Århus, Societas Ethica, 2003, pp. 101-112.

JOHN PAUL II, *Evangelium Vitae*, Encyclical Letter on the Value and Inviolability of Human Life, Rome, 25 March 1995.

KENNEDY, J., *Een weloverwogen dood. Euthanasie in Nederland* [A well-considered death. Euthanasia in the Netherlands], Amsterdam, Bert Bakker, 2002.

KÖRTNER, U.H.J., 'Therapieverzicht am Lebensende? Ethische Fragen des medizinischen assistierten Sterbens' in *Zeitschrift für medizinischen Ethik* 48(2002), pp. 15-28.

LEGET, C., *Ruimte om te sterven. Een weg voor zieken, naasten en zorgverleners* [Space to die. A path for patients, proxies and caregivers], Tielt, Lannoo, 2003.

MORCINIEC, P. (ed.), *Eutanazja w diskusji — Euthanasie in der Diskussion*, Opole, Wydzial Teologiczny, 2001.

RÖMELT, J., 'Autonomie und Sterben. Reicht eine Ethik der Selbstbestimmung zur Humanisierung des Todes?' in *Zeitschrift für medizinischen Ethik* 48(2002), pp. 3-14.

SECOND VATICAN COUNCIL, *Dignitatis Humanae Personae*, Declaration on Religious Freedom, Rome, 7 December 1965.

VAN DER WAL, G., A. VAN DER HEIDE, B.D. ONWUTEAKA-PHILIPSEN & P.J. VAN DER MAAS, *Medische besluitvorming aan het einde van het leven. De praktijk en de toetsingsprocedure euthanasie* [Medical decisionmaking at the end of life. Euthanasia procedure and review procedure], Utrecht, De Tijdstroom, 2003.

WOLBERT, W., *Du sollst nicht töten. Systematische Überlegungen zum Tötungsverbot*, Freiburg i. Br., Herder, 2000.

CARING FOR A DIGNIFIED END OF LIFE IN A CHRISTIAN HEALTH CARE INSTITUTION. THE VIEW OF CARITAS CATHOLICA FLANDERS

Chris Gastmans

Immediately following the approval of the Belgian Euthanasia Act, 'Caritas Catholica Flanders' sent a position paper to all affiliated institutions in which its standpoint regarding care for a dignified end of life is clarified. The ethical recommendations make explicit how medical and nursing expertise could effectively be employed in the interdisciplinary care context, so that the competent, terminally ill patient who requests euthanasia receives the best human care available. We would like to sketch very briefly the context in which this position paper should be placed, before reproducing the complete text of the recommendation.

1. General Background

'Caritas Catholica Flanders' (founded in 1932 at the behest of the Belgian bishops) is an umbrella organization for cooperation and consultation between the 'Association of Care Institutions' ('Verbond der Verzorgingsinstellingen'), grouping health-care institutions and services, and the 'Flemish Association for Public Welfare' ('Vlaams Welzijnsverbond'), grouping welfare institutions and services. The Association of Care Institutions is responsible for 62 general hospitals, 94 mental-health institutions and 326 geriatric-care institutions. The 'Flemish Association for Public Welfare' groups 397 facilities for handicapped persons and 344 facilities for public welfare (youth assistance, family support, child care and volunteer organizations).

In the past 70 years, Caritas has been a family inspired by a Christian anthropology and concept of care. This view cannot be construed as something fixed, something that could be copied and transmitted unchanged in all circumstances and for all times. To the contrary, the concept of the person and the idea of care that inspires the Caritas institutions must be continually refined and developed. Particularly the new ethical questions confronting those working in welfare and health care are an enormous challenge to the Christian viewpoint. For Caritas Flanders, this focus on ethical issues has gradually become a constant in its day-to-day operations.[1] The ethical interest is primarily manifested in the working of the two ethics committees linked to the Association of Care Institutions and the Flemish Association for Public Welfare. The task of the ethics committees is to provide orientation on the basis of a contemporary interpretation of a Christian anthropology and concept of care, and to help us deal responsibly with today's ethical questions.

The ethical recommendations contained in the document *Care for a dignified end of life* were drafted by the ethics committee of the Association of Care Institutions.[2] The committee began preparing the recommendations in January 2000 after six senators from the government coalition had, on 20 December 1999, submitted a joint legislative proposal concerning euthanasia to the Belgian senate. Another fact that urged the development of these recommendations, was the publication in November 2000 of a nationwide survey, wherein it was observed and estimated that 640 deaths in Flanders in 1998 resulted from euthanasia.[3] The debate on euthanasia and the research findings led Caritas Flanders to believe that caregivers will increasingly be confronted with euthanasia requests and will therefore be more involved in care for these patients.

---

[1] The prominent attention given by Caritas Flanders to ethical questions can also be illustrated by the international conference *Between technology and humanity: the impact of technology on health care ethics*, 18-19 October 2002, Brussels, organized on the occasion of Caritas Flanders's 70th anniversary. See C. GASTMANS (ed.), *Between Technology and Humanity: The Impact of Technology on Health Care Ethics*, Leuven, Leuven University Press, 2002.

[2] Other ethical recommendations drafted in recent years by the ethics committee of the 'Association of Care Institutions': *Choices in health care* (1996); *Termination of pregnancy* (1998); *Charging supplements in hospitals* (1998); *Evaluating protocols for drug research* (1999); *Artificial administration of food and fluids in the late terminal phase in demented patients* (2000); *Withholding or withdrawing life-prolonging medical treatment in the terminal phase* (2002); *Pluralism and ethical dialogue in Christian health care institutions* (2003).

[3] L. DELIENS *et al.*, 'End-of-life Decisions in Medical Practice in Flanders, Belgium' in *The Lancet* 356(2000), pp. 1806-1811.

The ethics committee's objective was to find an ethically well-founded answer to the question of how a Christian care institution should best ensure a dignified end of life. At the forefront was the fact that Belgium was close to approving the law on euthanasia. In developing these recommendations, the committee hoped to make a constructive contribution to serious opinion formation and construction of a position regarding end-of-life care among the employees of local care institutions. In no sense was it the intention to give these recommendations a compulsory or mandatory character. The ethical recommendations indicate standpoints, contain interpretations, refer to missing elements, place accents, make suggestions for improving the quality of decision-making with regard to the end of life — but there are no prohibitions. Indeed, any prohibition would run counter to the nature and intent of an ethical 'recommendation' or background text.

After extensive discussion (from January 2000 to May 2002) within the ethics committee of the Association of Care Institutions, and following numerous consultations with experts in terminal care for patients, the board of directors of Caritas Flanders approved the recommendations. On 17 May 2002, the day after the Belgian parliament passed the law on euthanasia, the Caritas recommendations were sent to its 1223 member institutions. For several months, the recommendations had been the focus of media commentary, both pro and con, by ethicists, lawyers, politicians, caregivers, etc., not infrequently in a polemical and unsubtle manner. Local care institutions of a Christian stamp use these recommendations as a reference document to develop ideas and policy regarding end-of-life care and put it into practice. In what follows, we indicate a number of ethical orientations for dealing responsibly with the euthanasia law in the Christian health-care institution, as they are recommended by Caritas Flanders.

2. Fundamental Choices

The starting point is the principle that everything possible should be done to provide support and assistance to the dying person and his or her family members, and to fulfil his or her wish for a dignified end of life. Before sketching the outlines of such care for a dignified end of life, a number of basic presuppositions regarding the human person and the value of autonomy must first be clarified.

2.1. *Respect for the human person*

Care providers are often confronted with problem situations in which the very dignity of the human person is in some way at stake. The Christian tradition has always maintained respect for the person as an ideal. The ethical demand for unconditional respect for one's fellow man is founded on the fact that we belong to the community of persons, that we feel connected with other persons and that the other must be recognized as such; it is also founded on the unique relation between God and man.

The unconditional affirmation of the dignity of the human person, understood as a relational being, is the point of departure for views endorsed by Caritas. Human dignity cannot be forfeited, not even through illness, handicap or an impending death. In other words, every person remains a person to the very end, and must be treated as such. Being a person — and the respect deriving from it — cannot be made dependent on the possession of specific capacities, for instance mental or intellectual abilities. Personhood is rooted in the fact that every person is a unique being (individual) who, in and through relations with other persons (relational) becomes more human and as such is part of the society as a whole (social).[4]

2.2. *The value of autonomy*

In the debate about the end of life, emphasis is often placed on the patient's autonomy as an important value. The starting point is that people themselves should be able to decide about their lives, without interference from others. On this view, autonomy is seen as a form of individual self-determination. Autonomy, conceived as self-determination, is the opposite of being subjected to the decisions of others.

For Caritas Flanders, the doctor-patient relationship is structured neither by simple individual self-determination nor by subjection to others. Preference is given not so much to deciding for oneself but to deciding together. Along these lines, it is possible to interpret the value of autonomy as active self-determination with the assistance and support of others (relational autonomy). This relation with others does not detract from the autonomy of the person;

---

[4] This characterization of the human person as an individual, relational and social being is drawn from the personalistic tradition in ethics. See L. JANSSENS, 'Artificial Insemination. Ethical Considerations' in *Louvain Studies* 8(1980-1981), pp. 3-29.

to the contrary, it is precisely a condition of such autonomy. A person is in charge of his or her life to the extent that, in his or her choices and actions, he or she identifies with a life-world and a life-history, manifest as a narrative of mutual solidarity among people.[5]

On this basis, Caritas Flanders criticizes the tendency in the euthanasia law to stress only one aspect of being human, *i.e.*, the freedom to make choices oneself, without interference from others. This one-sided emphasis on autonomy as individual self-determination does an injustice to the human being in its totality. In addition to a conception of the person as an individual who expresses his or her autonomous decisions, Caritas Flanders believes the person should also be conceived in his or her relations with others (being human is being a fellow human) and in his or her responsible participation in the human community (social responsibility).

Contrary to the proponents of an individualistic view of the human person in which autonomy and care for others can scarcely be reconciled, Caritas Flanders opts for a conception of autonomy in which an integral role is ascribed to the relation between people, in terms of solidarity and responsibility. In this way, one can do justice to the fact that, in the final phase of their lives, people often go through an entire process in which they must constantly make hundreds of small and large decisions designed to make the end of their lives more dignified. To a significant extent, this process is based on a balance between autonomy and mutual dependence, not only on individual self-determination.[6] Vulnerable dependence and self-assured autonomy must be recognized as equal and mutually interwoven aspects of human existence. This interpretation of autonomy as a value that can only develop fully in a relational context takes account of the fact that there are always degrees of autonomy (no one is ever fully autonomous) and that people make choices in consultation with others. Also, this relational grounding of autonomy avoids people being forced into lonely isolation with the argument that

---

[5] The concept of 'relational autonomy' is currently the focus of theoretical work in the ethics of care. See C. MACKENZIE & N. STOLJAR (eds.), *Relational Autonomy: Feminist Perspectives on Autonomy, Agency, and the Social Self*, New York — Oxford, Oxford University Press, 2000.

[6] G. WIDDERSHOVEN, *Ethiek in de kliniek: Hedendaagse benaderingen in de ethiek van de gezondheidszorg* [Clinical ethics. Contemporary approaches in health ethics], Amsterdam, Boom, 2000.

"he himself chose it". The relational conception of autonomy implies that people assume responsibility for one another.

The Belgian euthanasia law justifies euthanasia primarily on the basis of the expressed will of a patient who requests to die in this manner. Caritas Flanders, on the other hand, claims that in addition to the patient's will (person-related condition), the medical and nursing criteria ('objective' or clinical conditions such as terminal state, the physical basis of pain and suffering, palliative alternatives, etc.) should also be part of the assessment, and there should be a balance between the patient's will and the medical or nursing criteria. Finding such a balance through common exploration and consultation between the patient, his/her loved ones, and the team of care providers offers the best guarantees for adequate protection of the human person as an autonomous individual, but also as a relational being.

Starting from these basic options with respect to the dignity of the human person and the value of relational autonomy, we now turn to a phased development of ethical directions concerning care for a dignified end of life. We deal in turn with palliative care, the decisions of physicians at the end of life, and the request for euthanasia.

3. Palliative Care For All

For Caritas Flanders, care for a dignified end of life deserves more attention in the Christian health-care institution. Concretely, this means that the development of a culture and structure for palliative care needs to be given the highest priority. When a cure is no longer possible, or when a disproportion arises between the effort required to keep someone alive and their dignity, then it is important to focus on ethically responsible and expert medical and nursing assistance to the dying person. The principles to be borne in mind, apart from the needs of every sick person — i.e., the need for security, dignity and physical comfort — are the patient's specific needs due to an approaching death: anxiety in the face of death, the need for answers to ultimate questions which dying people are inevitably confronted with, the need for closeness and relations with loved ones. The latter also need clear information and psychological and social support, so that they are able to carry out their role of being present at the end of life.

Every dying person has the right to expert medical and nursing assistance, in the framework of dignified integral care (bodily, mental, social and existential). One should expect that Christian healthcare institutions recognize this right and incorporate it into their mission statement. The recognition of this basic right can best be ensured by setting up a structure and a culture of palliative care.

The ethics committee supports the general opinion that good palliative care is considered to be a *sine qua non* of euthanasia, for the problem of the control of suffering still remains.[7] What then should be done? The first thing to do is to try to prevent the occurrence of those situations for which euthanasia has been suggested, by anticipating their onset and forestalling their development.[8] The second thing is to make available to terminal patients all the methods of relief and control of distressing symptoms which are now available.[9] Finally, it must be recognized that the care of the patient and the relief of his or her suffering are never purely medical concerns, and so we must provide for their physical, mental, and spiritual well-being by involving all the caring professions in an effective and sensitive approach to the patient and his or her family in order to support them in their situation of need.[10] For this reason, the consulting physician should at an early stage appeal to the expertise of a specialized palliative support team in order to discuss the palliative possibilities and to apply them in a way that alleviates the patient's suffering as much as possible.

When it becomes clear that a terminal patient's pain and distress cannot adequately be combated using 'normal' palliative methods,

---

[7] B. Onwuteaka-Philipsen & G. van der Wal, 'A Protocol for Consultation of Another Physician in Cases of Euthanasia and Assisted Suicide' in *Journal of Medical Ethics* 27(2001), pp. 331-337; T. Quill, B. Lo & D. Brock, 'Palliative Options of Last resort: A Comparison of Voluntary Stopping Eating and Drinking, Terminal Sedation, Physician-Assisted Suicide, and Voluntary Active Euthanasia' in *Journal of the American Medical Association* 278(1997), pp. 2099-2104; B. Broeckaert & R. Janssens, 'Palliative Care and Euthanasia: Belgian and Dutch Perspectives' in this volume, pp. 35-69.

[8] D. Doyle, G. Hanks & N. MacDonald (eds.), *Oxford Textbook of Palliative Medicine*, 2nd ed., Oxford, Oxford University Press, 1998.

[9] *Ibid.*

[10] H.M. Chochinov, 'Dignity-Conserving Care: A New Model for Palliative Care' in *Journal of the American Medical Association* 287(2002), pp. 2253-2260; W. Breithart *et al.*, 'Depression, Hopelessness, and Desire for Hastened Death in Terminally Ill Patients with Cancer' in *Journal of American Medical Assocation* 284(2000), pp. 2907-2911.

the technique of palliative sedation could be taken into consideration.[11] In the context of palliative care, palliative sedation refers to "the intentional administration of sedative drugs in dosages and combinations required to reduce the consciousness of a terminal patient as much as necessary to adequately relieve one or more refractory symptoms".[12] Palliative sedation is only considered when one is confronted with a refractory symptom which causes the patient enormous suffering and prevents a dignified death. A symptom can be considered refractory to treatment when it cannot be adequately controlled in spite of every tolerable effort to provide relief within an acceptable time period without compromising consciousness.[13] The most frequent reasons for inducing sedation are delirium, dyspnea and pain[14], but also psychological symptoms can be considered as refractory.

The experience of palliative support teams shows that such an active and integral approach (palliative care including palliative sedation) can, in many cases, displace the euthanasia request and allow the patient to die in a dignified manner without euthanasia. This means that Christian health-care institutions should conceive of palliative care as an active and integral approach employed in the case of *every terminal patient*, rather than seeing it as one alternative alongside euthanasia.

Caritas Flanders believes that it would be desirable, if at all possible, for terminal patients to remain in familiar surroundings until they die. The obvious solution is therefore to contribute to supporting initiatives that will provide genuine help to patients who want to pass their final months at home or in an environment that substitutes

[11] J. PORTA, 'Palliative Sedation: Clinical Aspects' in C. GASTMANS (ed.), *Between Technology and Humanity: The Impact of Technology on Health Care Ethics*, Leuven: Leuven University Press, 2002, pp. 219-237; B. BROECKAERT & J.-M. NUÑEZ OLARTE, 'Sedation in Palliative Care: Facts and Concepts' in H. TEN HAVE & D. CLARKE (eds.), *The Ethics of Palliative Care: European Perspectives*, Buckingham, Open University Press, 2002, pp. 166-180.

[12] J. PORTA, 'Palliative Sedation: Clinical Aspects' in C. GASTMANS (ed.), *Between Technology and Humanity: The Impact of Technology on Health Care Ethics*, Leuven, Leuven University Press, 2002, pp. 219-237; B. BROECKAERT & J.-M. NUÑEZ OLARTE, 'Sedation in Palliative Care: Facts and Concepts' in H. TEN HAVE & D. CLARKE (eds.), *The Ethics of Palliative Care: European Perspectives*, Buckingham, Open University Press, 2002, pp. 166-180.

[13] *Ibid.*

[14] J. PORTA, 'Terminal Sedation: A Review of the Clinical Literature' in *European Journal of Palliative Care* 8(2001), pp. 97-100.

for a home. To this end, health-care institutions would do well, among other things, to improve their cooperation with specialized palliative home care teams, who can carefully prepare the patient's return home. Elderly people who live in a nursing home should be able to stay there until the end of their lives. Hospitalization in this phase should be avoided as much as possible.

To sum up, we could say that Christian health-care institutions have the important task of developing the palliative support team into an interdisciplinary advisory and assistance team for palliative care and end-of-life counselling. The palliative support team can sensitize and train the medical and paramedical personnel, can give advice on symptom and pain control, can lend their support in difficult cases (*e.g.*, in cases of palliative sedation) and in making preparations for the patient to return home, to go to a nursing home, or for a transfer to a residential unit of palliative care. They could even receive such patients temporarily themselves, if need be. Finally, the palliative support team plays a crucial role with respect to patients who request, or persist in requesting euthanasia.

4. The Ethical Quality of End-of-Life Decisions in Medical Practice

Euthanasia (the administration of lethal drugs with the explicit intention of shortening the patient's life at the patient's explicit request) cannot be considered in isolation from the entire set of end-of-life decisions in medical practice. By end-of-life decisions we understand life-terminating action (euthanasia, physician-assisted suicide, termination of life without the patient's explicit request), alleviation of pain and symptoms with opioids in doses with a potential life-shortening effect (pain control, palliative sedation) and withholding or withdrawing potential life-prolonging treatment (*e.g.*, withdrawing artificial food and fluid administration).[15]

It is of utmost importance that the decision-making regarding the end-of-life decisions just mentioned be accompanied by as much openness and communication as possible among the parties involved: the dying patient, his or her loved ones, the physicians

---

[15] L. DELIENS *et al.*, 'End-of-life Decisions in Medical Practice in Flanders, Belgium' in *The Lancet* 356(2000), pp. 1806-1811.

responsible, the nurses and paramedics. After all, these are not purely 'medical' but also 'ethical' decisions. Questions of dignity and meaningfulness transcend the medical-technical discourse and require an ethical judgement in which all parties can enter into dialogue on an equal footing.

Following the Belgian Order of Physicians' code of conduct (cf. art. 33, 96 and 97), it is recommended that clear procedures be established regarding the way in which clinical-ethical decision-making is carried out in these matters. The pursuit of transparent, open communication among members of the medical and nursing teams, providing well-measured doses of information to the patient and his/her loved ones in order to permit informed free consent — these are just a few of the conditions that must be fulfilled in such delicate decision-making processes. Finally, one must ensure that this decision-making is not infected by arguments of a financial or economic nature. In many cases, the general practitioner can fulfil an important role in reaching a consensus among all parties concerned.

In developing such procedures, the local ethics committees within the hospitals also have a significant role to play. They can also establish concrete procedures for specific patient groups, for instance demented geriatric patients, terminal patients, patients in a persistent vegetative state, etc.[16]

Something should also be said about the so-called emergency cases, in which the support team is suddenly and unexpectedly confronted with a patient in extreme distress and where immediate decisions must be made without the possibility of following the normal decision-making procedure (interdisciplinary consultations, informed consent, etc.). We have in mind emergency patients following a fire or traffic accident where the victims have experienced extremely painful burns and find themselves in a hopeless state where they can no longer be helped. In such cases, the euthanasia law passed by the Belgian parliament offers the physician no legal security nor even any legitimation. If a physician ends the life of a

---

[16] See *e.g.* C. GASTMANS, 'Tube Feeding and Assisted Oral Feeding in Demented Patients with Eating Difficulties: A Clinical Ethical Approach' in C. GASTMANS (ed.), *Between Technology and Humanity: The Impact of Technology on Health Care Ethics*, Leuven, Leuven University Press, 2002, pp. 197-216; BRITISH MEDICAL ASSOCIATION, *Withholding and Withdrawing Life Prolonging Medical Treatment: Guidance for Decision Making*, London, BMJ Books, 2001.

patient in such a predicament then he or she will be subject to prosecution and will have to answer to the judicial authorities. Nevertheless it is a form of euthanasia that can be ethically justified. What is more, in this case one can recognize a type of euthanasia that has been legitimate for centuries on the basis of medical urgency.

5. Euthanasia and Terminally Ill Patients

5.1. *When termination of life is requested*

In some cases the patient makes a request for euthanasia and clearly makes it known that he or she would like to die in this manner. Care providers faced with a request for euthanasia must at least be willing to listen carefully to the request, which means that there must be an opportunity for the feelings of the patient, and those of the patient's loved ones, to be aired, as well as their uncertainties and practical questions. Patients who request euthanasia must be able to count on an adequate reception from the medical team, the nurses and the other care providers (psychologist, pastoral counsellor, etc.), in which approachability and assistance are central factors. It would be contrary to the aforementioned guidelines concerning care for a dignified end of life if such a request were to be ignored by the physician when medical decision-making takes place. On the other hand however, the conception of relational autonomy outlined above gives rise to the question whether the patient's request is by itself a necessary but not sufficient reason for initiating euthanasia.

In cases where a competent patient repeatedly makes a euthanasia request, the physician's responsibility cannot be limited to listening sympathetically to the suffering patient. The Belgian Euthanasia Act (art. 3 §2 1°) stipulates that the physician must inform the patient of the possibility of palliative care. Caritas Flanders would like to emphasize — even more than the legislation does — the importance of adequately implementing palliative possibilities. The development of the 'palliative filter' procedure represents an important ethical benefit in caring for patients at the end of life.

5.2. *The palliative filter procedure*

The physician is expected to employ every resource to determine whether the patient's request is grounded in an autonomous, free and informed choice. In other words, the physician must see whether it is not actually a so-called pseudo-request for euthanasia.[17] To this end, the following procedure is proposed.

The physician will:
- on the basis of the patient's medical file thoroughly investigate the concrete possibilities for palliative care (including palliative sedation) and its consequences in consultation with the hospital's palliative support team or with the local consultative structure for palliative care;
- fully inform the patient about all aspects of his/her health situation and about the various existing possibilities for palliative care and its consequences. In these cases, the patient will be provided with the palliative support team's recommendations and the patient will explicitly be given an opportunity to consult the palliative support team, should he or she so desire, and discuss the concrete possibilities for palliative care and its consequences;
- ensure that the patient is given an opportunity to discuss his or her request with any person of his/her choosing, including the nursing team with which the patient is in regular contact;
- thoroughly discuss the euthanasia request, and the patient's situation, with the nursing team;
- if the patient so desires, discuss the euthanasia request with such friends and family as the patient designates;
- lend support to the patient's friends and family.

The procedure just described guarantees that all terminal patients will be offered good palliative care. Caritas Flanders believes that this 'palliative filter' will in the first instance work as a preventive measure with respect to euthanasia requests.

5.3. *If the euthanasia request persists*

Caritas Flanders acknowledges that despite a careful implementation of the palliative filter procedure, the physician and other members of the support team may, in rare and exceptional cases, be faced with a

---

[17] B. BROECKAERT, 'Goede zorg voor de dood: Palliatieve consultatie bij elk verzoek om euthanasie [Optimal care before dying. Palliative consult for every euthanasia request]' in *Medisch contact* 55/45(2000), pp. 1597-1600; B. BROECKAERT, 'Voor een efficiënte en zinvolle euthanasieprocedure [For an efficient and meaningful euthanasia procedure]' in *Palliatieve zorg* 7/4(2000), p. 3 and p. 16.

conflict of conscience when the patient's suffering (and the euthanasia request deriving from it) does not diminish. It is precisely here that one's conscience has the important task of weighing alternatives, guided on the one hand by fundamental values such as respect for the patient's autonomy and respect for life, and on the other hand by judging how these values can best emerge from the conflict in question. In these cases, Caritas Flanders respects a decision made in good conscience by the physician and members of the support team to initiate euthanasia, assuming that the physician opts for the most humane choice possible.[18] In these specific circumstances, the most humane choice consists in finding a balance among values that express respect for human dignity. In concrete terms, this means that a balance must be struck between the will of the patient and the result of checking the euthanasia request against clinical criteria (including whether the situation is terminal, the physical grounding of suffering, palliative alternatives, etc.).

In these extremely difficult circumstances, the palliative team must make an effort to preserve human dignity as much as possible. Prerequisites for an actual decision to initiate euthanasia are:
– that the request comes from a mentally competent, terminally ill patient who has attained the age of majority;
– that it is an explicit, voluntary, unambiguous, well-considered, repeated and sustainable request (as determined by the palliative filter procedure described above);
– that the process of dying has already begun (*i.e.*, terminal phase);
– that there exist sufficiently serious medical reasons for considering the request to initiate euthanasia, *i.e.*, irremediable and severe suffering based on a physical cause, and a medically futile terminal situation.

Caritas Flanders would like to stress that the application of these minimal criteria should be part of a more global approach to care for a dignified end of life, as it has been elaborated here. It is therefore utterly unacceptable to view these guidelines outside their overall context and use them as the sole conditions for dealing with a euthanasia request. Likewise it bears repeating that, in accordance with the views already elaborated concerning 'relational autonomy',

---

[18] Paul Schotsmans during the public hearings in the Belgian Senate, 22 February 2000.

decision-making with regard to euthanasia should take place in and through dialogue.

6. Euthanasia and Non-Terminally Ill Patients

Although it is difficult to formulate a conclusive definition of the so-called terminal phase, Caritas Flanders believes that the choice for euthanasia can only be considered in the context of the terminal phase of illness. Euthanasia is only appropriate in situations where death is expected within a foreseeable length of time (hours, days or weeks), where the process of dying is already underway. In the past, euthanasia has always been connected to a patient who is in the terminal phase.

Moreover, for Caritas Flanders euthanasia is only relevant in situations of unbearable physical suffering (or suffering caused by a process of physical degeneration) for which medical remedies can be sought. Purely mental or existential distress does not fall into this category.

The physician is only confronted with a crisis of conscience when he/she is faced with a situation where he/she would like to help the patient with his/her medical expertise, but the medical resources at his/her disposal are no longer sufficient to alleviate the physically based suffering of the terminal patient.[19] The objective nature of the conditions of terminality, intolerability and untreatability (where a physical cause lies at the basis) is generally accepted as a decisive argument for rejecting euthanasia in non-terminal patients and for purely mental or existential distress.[20]

For Caritas Flanders, the situation of non-terminal patients and patients suffering from purely mental or existential distress falls outside the euthanasia problematic. Caritas Flanders regrets that the Belgian euthanasia law as approved does not draw a clear distinction between euthanasia and assisted suicide. We would like to stress that society has a responsibility to care for this group of patients. The impact of life-shortening action in non-terminal patients is too unreasonably large to consider it as an ethically permissible practice.

---

[19] Fernand Van Neste during the public hearings in the Belgian Senate, 15 February 2000.

[20] M. GUNDERSON & D. MAYO, 'Restricting Physician-Assisted Death to the Terminally Ill' in *Hastings Center Report* 30/6(2000), pp. 17-23.

Care providers must give these patients a guarantee that they will be able to resort to the best possible quality of care, and that they will not be in any way shortchanged. Society must create room to expand and guarantee quality care for these persons.[21]

7. Euthanasia, Incompetent Patients and Advance Directives

A special problem that cannot be left out of the discussion here is care for a dignified end of life in incompetent patients. By incompetent patients, we mean persons in a state where they can no longer express their will about decisions regarding their own persons (health, treatment, bodily integrity, quality of life, dying with dignity, etc.). For the benefit of incompetent persons, the euthanasia law provides a legal basis for the so-called advance directive. Caritas Flanders regrets that, in the Belgian law, the scope of an advance directive is restricted exclusively to *active termination of life*. We employ a broader conception of the advance directive: it is a written document in which a person, preceding the onset of his/her incompetence, gives specific instructions regarding the medical decisions that he/she wishes to be made, and designates a possible contact person whom the physician must consult when taking any end-of-life decision about the incompetent person.

The advance directive (and the contact person) can be a valuable element when the care team must take a decision about a dignified end of life for incompetent persons. Such an advance directive gives the patient the possibility of making his/her opinion known on issues such as therapeutic obstinacy, inhumane situations, disproportional (unreasonable) treatments, an so on. The advance directive can offer the patient greater psychological comfort. It also provides the physician with additional information to be included in the broad decision-making process in which the patient's loved ones and the care team also take part. For Caritas Flanders, however, it is important that such an expression of one's will is also accompanied, as much as possible, by the designation of a contact person who has the patient's trust, someone who can discuss therapeutic choices with the

---

[21] Paul Schotsmans during the public hearings in the Belgian Senate, 22 February 2000.

physician and the care team. Moreover, the contact person can continue the dialogue established between the care team and the patient in a way which, though imperfect, can nevertheless be considered significant.

Given the possible difficulties associated with interpreting an advance directive, and in light of the extreme position of weakness occupied by an incompetent patient and the exceptionally delicate (and irreversible) nature of action to end life, Caritas Flanders recommends a cautious and restrictive application of the advance directive (and contact person). The advance directive (and contact person) should be used to allow the patient to die in as dignified a manner as possible, without transgressing the border of therapeutic obstinacy or intentionally life-ending action.

In concrete terms, this means that in cases of medical action that has become futile, the choice should be to completely discontinue all medical therapy. Caritas Flanders emphasizes that decision-making with regard to withdrawing medical therapy must occur within well-structured consultations and must go together with appropriate nursing care (general bodily hygiene, care for the patient's comfort, care for wounds, etc.). Expert palliative support must ensure that the patient's human dignity, despite extreme degeneration, is respected as much as possible.

Caritas Flanders unambiguously stresses the ethical unacceptability of intentionally ending the life of an incompetent patient who has never drafted an advance directive (whether or not the patient had the opportunity to do so). The sole ethical criterion that the physician and nursing team must employ is to aim at the best possible quality of life (or death) for the patient concerned. Here again, in cases of medical action that has become futile, the choice should be to completely withdraw all medical therapy.

8. Some Specific Points of Concern Relating to Decision-Making

Many parties are always involved in decision-making regarding the end of life. Besides the patient and his/her relatives, the physician, the nurses (and in some cases other care providers such as a psychologist or pastoral counsellor), and the health-care institution play a role. It is essential that the emotional reactions, intuitions and viewpoints of all parties are taken seriously. This can better be achieved within a model of open communication than with an approach where individual self-determination is predominant. Communication involves taking account of the other's point of view. This can also be done through exhibiting silent attention.[22]

8.1. *The patient and his/her relatives*

It is essential for the success of the palliative filter procedure that the patient and his/her loved ones are motivated from the outset to participate in a process of exploring together the possible courses of action. The underlying idea is that it cannot be objectively determined in advance what is best in a given situation, but that this can only be discovered by relating various different points of view on the matter (the views of the palliative support team, the patient and his/her loved ones, the care team, etc.). This communication process can identify possible pseudo-questions and pseudo-solutions (based on incomplete or inaccurate information).

For Caritas Flanders, decision-making regarding the end of life cannot be conceived as a one-off act by an individual (*e.g.*, a patient who demands euthanasia with no further discussion), but as a process of interpersonal agreement (patient, loved ones, care team and palliative support team who enter into a dialogue prompted by a euthanasia request). The ideas of the various parties in this decision-making process are not considered to be fixed facts leading to immediate action, but as the object of communal exploration and discussion.[23] This process-oriented approach does not mean that the patient's will is unimportant. The patient's wishes are crucial, but in many cases (especially the first requests for euthanasia) they cannot be formulated simply. In many cases, the precise content of the patient's will must be explored and further refined, even for the patient him/herself. So the patient's will cannot replace dialogue. To the contrary, it is only through common exploration and deliberation that the patient's genuine will can gradually become clear. For this reason, interpersonal dialogue can be seen as an essential form of respect for the patient's will (and hence the patient's relational autonomy). It is then not an individual claim to autonomy, but an autonomy shared in common.

---

[22] G. WIDDERSHOVEN, *Ethiek in de kliniek: Hedendaagse benaderingen in de ethiek van de gezondheidszorg* [Clinical ethics. Contemporary approaches in health care ethics], Amsterdam, Boom, 2000.

[23] *Ibid.*

8.2. *The nursing team*

Due to the intertwining of both medical and nursing aspects in care for a dignified end of life, it is essential that physicians and nurses (and other care providers such as psychologists and pastoral counsellors) arrive at good cooperative relations, with respect for one another's contribution.

The patient's request for euthanasia will not always, or not in the first instance, be directed to the physician: usually it is directed to the nurse.[24] In this initial phase, the nurse's specific task includes being receptive to the signals that might contain a wish to die and communicating this information to the physician (unless the patient explicitly forbids this). In this phase, it is also important for the nurse to carefully observe and assist the patient, for instance by paying close attention to how the patient emotionally processes information. The nurse must also be attuned to the relations and the discussions with the patient's friends and family.

If the physician is the first one to be confronted with the euthanasia request, he/she should follow the guideline that this request should be discussed with the members of the nursing team who are directly involved in caring for the patient (again, unless the patient explicitly forbids this).

When a nurse is involved in directly caring for a patient who makes a euthanasia request, he/she must participate in the decision-making process that accompanies the "palliative filter" procedure, since the nurse's daily involvement and his/her specific expertise mean that he/she will be able to make a significant contribution to finding a solution to the patient's request. Caritas Flanders emphatically supports close cooperation between all professional care providers. General practitioners can also play an important role here.

Ultimate responsibility for all end-of-life decisions rests with the physician, because of his/her medical expertise and his/her legal competence.

The dying patient has the right to direct a euthanasia request to any care provider, but in this case the same principle that applies to any request for help is valid: one cannot deny the care provider the

---

[24] A. VAN DER SCHEUR & A. VAN DER AREND, 'The Role of the Nurse in Euthanasia: A Dutch Study' in *Nursing Ethics* 5(1998), pp. 497-508; T. DE BEER, C. GASTMANS & B. DIERCKX DE CASTERLÉ, 'Involvement of Nurses in Euthanasia: A Review of the Literature' in *Journal of Medical Ethics* 30(2004), pp. 494-498.

right to follow his/her conscience. On the grounds of principled objections, a physician or nurse has the right not to take part in the decision-making or the administration of euthanasia. However, every care provider does have a duty to listen to the patient's euthanasia request and to take any steps necessary to ensure an adequate implementation of the "palliative filter" procedure.

8.3. *The health-care institution*

Given the complexity of the decision-making and the diversity of professional backgrounds among the parties involved, Caritas Flanders urges the hospital's local ethics committee to formulate recommendations concerning care for a dignified end of life. In so doing, explicit attention should be given to dealing with euthanasia requests. In addition, guidelines should be formulated that facilitate smooth implementation of the "palliative filter" procedure. Caritas Flanders does not anticipate the direct participation of members of the local ethics committee in the clinical decision-making regarding the end of life, unless the care providers request this explicitly.

Caritas Flanders would like to remind the Christian hospitals that they have the right, on the basis of their religious identity, to formulate an ethical policy that will orient care for a dignified end of life within their institution. On this point, hospitals can come to an understanding with their staff physicians.

It is not enough to spell out guidelines on care for a dignified end of life. It is also important that this policy is made known inside and outside the hospital walls, so that prospective patients and (prospective) staff members know what they might expect. A mission statement and a patient brochure offer many possibilities in this respect.[25]

Conclusion

Care that ensures a dignified end of life deserves more attention from care providers and from society at large. In this position paper, Caritas Flanders has shown that care for a dignified end of life is not

---

[25] I. HAVERKATE *et al.*, 'Guidelines on Euthanasia and Pain Alleviation: Compliance and Opinions of Physicians' in *Health Policy* 44(1998), pp. 45-55.

something that stands on its own. For instance, the question of how care providers should deal with euthanasia requests is closely related to our views about the human person and about the place of autonomy in people's lives. The problem of euthanasia is also an issue within the overall approach to palliative care and end-of-life decisions in medical practice. In this position paper, Caritas Flanders has illustrated why the problematic surrounding the end of life cannot be 'solved' using a purely medical approach. Perhaps the very suggestion that there can be a solution is already misguided. If we consider the issue carefully, it is clear that the death of people is not something to be 'solved', but something that can only be given a more or less suitable form. There is probably no form that will be acceptable to everyone. The form outlined here is an appeal, from a Christian perspective, to all those who work in Christian health-care institutions to develop a strong ethical awareness regarding end-of-life care.

References

BREITBART, W., B. ROSENFELD, H. PESSIN, M. KAIM, J. FUNESTI-ESCH, M. GALIETTA, C. NELSON & R. BRESCIA, 'Depression, Hopelessness, and Desire for Hastened Death in Terminally Ill Patients with Cancer' in *Journal of American Medical Association* 284(2000), pp. 2907-2911.

BRITISH MEDICAL ASSOCIATION, *Withholding and Withdrawing Life Prolonging Medical Treatment: Guidance for Decision Making*, London, BMJ Books, 2001.

BROECKAERT, B., 'Goede zorg voor de dood: Palliatieve consultatie bij elk verzoek om euthanasie [Optimal care before dying. Palliative consult for every euthanasia request]' in *Medisch contact* 55/45(2000), pp. 1597-1600.

BROECKAERT, B., 'Voor een efficiënte en zinvolle euthanasieprocedure [For an efficient and meaningful euthanasiaprocedure]' in *Palliatieve zorg* 7/4 (2000), p. 3 and p. 16.

BROECKAERT, B. & J.-M. NUÑEZ OLARTE, 'Sedation in Palliative Care: Facts and Concepts' in H. TEN HAVE & D. CLARKE, *The Ethics of Palliative Care: European Perspectives*, Buckingham, Open University Press, 2002, pp. 166-180.

CHOCHINOV, H.M., 'Dignity-Conserving Care: A New Model for Palliative Care' in *Journal of the American Medical Association* 287(2002), pp. 2253-2260.

De Beer, T., C. Gastmans & B. Dierckx de Casterlé, 'Involvement of Nurses in Euthanasia: A Review of the Literature' in *Journal of Medical Ethics* 30(2004), pp. 494-498.

Deliens, L., F. Mortier, J. Bilsen, M. Cosyns, R. Vander Stichele, J. Vanoverloop, & K. Ingels, 'End-of-life Decisions in Medical Practice in Flanders, Belgium' in *The Lancet* 356(2000), pp. 1806-1811.

Doyle, D., G. Hanks & N. MacDonald (eds.), *Oxford Textbook of Palliative Medicine*, 2nd ed., Oxford, Oxford University Press, 1998.

Gastmans, C., 'Tube Feeding and Assisted Oral Feeding in Demented Patients with Eating Difficulties: A Clinical Ethical Approach' in C. Gastmans (ed.), *Between Technology and Humanity: The Impact of Technology on Health Care Ethics*, Leuven, Leuven University Press, 2002, pp. 197-216.

Haverkate, I., G. van der Wal, P. van der Maas, B. Onwuteaka-Philipsen & P. Kostense, 'Guidelines on Euthanasia and Pain Alleviation: Compliance and Opinions of Physicians' in *Health Policy* 44(1998), pp. 45-55.

Janssens, L., 'Artificial Insemination. Ethical Considerations' in *Louvain Studies* 8(1980-1981), pp. 3-29.

Mackenzie, C. & N. Stoljar (eds.), *Relational Autonomy: Feminist Perspectives on Autonomy, Agency, and the Social Self*, New York — Oxford, Oxford University Press, 2000.

Onwuteaka-Philipsen, B. & G. van der Wal, 'A Protocol for Consultation of Another Physician in Cases of Euthanasia and Assisted Suicide' in *Journal of Medical Ethics* 27(2001), pp. 331-337.

Porta, J., 'Palliative Sedation: Clinical Aspects' in C. Gastmans (ed.), *Between Technology and Humanity: The Impact of Technology on Health Care Ethics*, Leuven, Leuven University Press, 2002, pp. 219-237.

Porta J., 'Terminal Sedation: A Review of the Clinical Literature' in *European Journal of Palliative Care* 8(2001), pp. 97-100.

Quill, T., B. Lo & D. Brock, 'Palliative Options of Last Resort: A Comparison of Voluntarily Stopping Eating and Drinking, Terminal Sedation, Physician-Assisted Suicide, and Voluntary Active Euthanasia' in *Journal of American Medical Association* 278(1997), pp. 2099-2104.

van der Scheur, A. & A. van der Arend, 'The Role of the Nurse in Euthanasia: A Dutch Study' in *Nursing Ethics* 5 (1998), pp. 497-508.

Widdershoven, G., *Ethiek in de kliniek: Hedendaagse benaderingen in de ethiek van de gezondheidszorg* [Clinical ethics. Contemporary approaches in health ethics], Amsterdam, Boom, 2000.

EUTHANASIA AND PLURALISM[1]

Herman De Dijn

1. What is pluralism?

It is gradually starting to sink in that there are two types of pluralism: a 'neutral' pluralism and an 'authentic' pluralism.[2] Those who support neutral pluralism believe that values and norms, especially as related to religious views or traditions, are personal matters which do not belong in the public arena or the political sphere. The ideal would be that even domains such as healthcare and education would be completely neutral as well. Healthcare professionals should in other words abstract from their personal views and values for the benefit of the patient. In this perspective, no healthcare or educational institution would be allowed to implement any selectivity with regard to its management, services or patients. When, in a society, the hold of religious groups on institutions compromises the achievement of this ideal, a pluralistic policy of dismantling monopolies and exclusiveness must be pursued. Often a deeply rooted aversion to any religious influence on society is behind this strategy — at least that's how things are in Belgium. Another reason for pursuing this policy is the expectation that, in this way, cohesion in society will be strengthened or, at least, that the impact of ideological oppositions in society will be reduced.

---

[1] This contribution is based on a lecture held during a workshop on 'Ethical policies on the subject of euthanasia' organised by the Faculty of Medicine (Catholic University of Leuven, Belgium) and the Association of Care Institutions on 6 February 2004, Leuven. My views concerning ethics, bioethics and applied ethics in general can be found in H. DE DIJN, *Taboes, monsters en loterijen. Ethiek in de laat-moderne tijd* [Taboos, monsters and lotteries. Ethics in the late modern era], Kapellen/Kampen, Pelckmans/Klement, 2003.

[2] See Internal Notice no. 8 (dd. 24 October 2003) of the VERBOND DER VERZORGINGS-INSTELLINGEN, entitled 'Pluralisme en ethische dialoog in christelijke verzorgingsinstellingen' [Association of Care Institutions, 'Pluralism and ethical dialogue in Christian healthcare institutions'].

'Authentic' pluralism (or 'real' pluralism as I will call it) implies that values and norms are not and cannot be merely personal matters but inevitably play an important role in the public and political sphere. So-called 'neutrality' is therefore illusory.[3] Furthermore, real pluralism holds that it is a *good* thing that values and norms play a role especially in fields such as healthcare, where highly sensitive matters that concern the very essence of human life are at stake. Patients do not want healthcare practice to be reduced to neutral technical operations but rather prefer it to be based on the specific values that are central to the healthcare institution's mission as traditionally understood.[4]

A second important distinction for our discussion is the difference between external and internal pluralism. In Belgium, defenders of real pluralism are confronted with the fact that religiously affiliated healthcare institutions attract a large group of patients precisely because of the combination of value orientation *and* professionalism. This success has led to a situation where a majority of care providers and patients feel little or no affinity with the religious origins and the related ethical positions that have for so long been the basis of Catholic healthcare institutions. Hence, the following paradox arises: patients continue to choose *en masse* Catholic institutions hoping to find quality care that is supported by a specific vocation, while that success itself makes it increasingly unlikely that in these institutions enough professionals operate from such a vocation.

The answer given within Catholic institutions to this confusing situation is expressed in the term 'internal pluralism'.[5] The central element of internal pluralism is the choice of an 'open dialogue' between the various value orientations that are supposed to be present in today's healthcare institutions. On the assumption that they recognise the promotion of human dignity, each value orientation must be able to maintain its own profile within the institution. Open dialogue should even lead to the strengthening of the identity of the

---

[3] See H. DE DIJN, 'Voorbij de ontzuiling [Beyond de-pillarisation]' in *Streven* 69/4(2002), pp. 301-311. See also H. DE DIJN, 'Cultural Identity, Religion, Moral Pluralism and the Law' in *Bijdragen. International Journal in Philosophy and Theology* 64/3(2003), pp. 286-298.

[4] H. DE DIJN, 'Voorbij de ontzuiling [Beyond de-pillarisation].'

[5] This term plays an important role in the Advice no. 8 of the Association of Care Institutions on pluralism and ethical dialogue (see footnote 2).

different sides. At the same time, a critical attitude towards the Christian ethical tradition should be assumed. Proponents of internal pluralism cherish the hope that the different views will not be weakened during the process of consensus building, for instance while drawing up the institution's mission statement or when ethical guidelines are formulated.

In the light of the current situation these seem to be very optimistic expectations with regard to internal pluralism. When pluralism is conceived in this way the question arises whether this will not *de facto* result in abandoning one's own orientation, thereby producing a situation of neutral pluralism. Internal pluralism would be required to cope with the presence of individuals who have radically different or even opposed values. However, at this post-modern juncture, many individuals have largely become estranged from *any* form of religion or philosophy of life, so the plea for internal pluralism may well veil a widespread philosophical indifference and 'post-modern tolerance'.[6]

As far as the open dialogue is concerned: how 'open' can that dialogue possibly be? Are all conclusions acceptable, including complete secularisation? What will be the role of, say, the ethics documents of the umbrella organization of Catholic healthcare institutions in the dialogue? How will the hitherto naturally privileged position of the Catholic pastoral service be approached within the institution? Why is it that a critical attitude is deemed necessary especially with respect to the Christian tradition and the ecclesiastical statements on ethics? Should it not rather be the case that one adopts a positive attitude and examines what the underlying reasons are for these views, instead of approaching them with a priori suspicion?[7] In any case, if one wishes to maintain at all the Christian character of a healthcare institution, it seems there can only be openness within certain limits, implying a dialogue undertaken under the strong guidance of a committed institutional management.

Anyone who has already been engaged in a dialogue concerning serious ethical problems with people who hold different beliefs or

---

[6] On 'postmodern tolerance' see H. DE DIJN, 'Tolerance, Loyalty to Values and Respect for the Law' in *Ethical Perspectives* 1/1(1994), pp. 27-32.

[7] The same problem occurs with fundamental religious concepts which, out of lack of understanding, are thrown overboard as hocus-pocus. A good example of this is 'original sin'. See H. SCHWALL, 'Erfzonde, erfwonde' in *TGL* (Tijdschrift voor Geestelijk Leven) 59/5(2003), pp. 529-541.

adhere to divergent value patterns knows how difficult it is to find a consensus. The differences of opinion within the Belgian Advisory Committee on Bio-ethics are a good example of this. It is an illusion to think that ethical viewpoints — even when defended by well-meaning discussion partners — can always be brought to a consensus which each participant can identify with. Fundamental ethical differences are at a different level than that of venting opinions or applying principles or rules in a discussion.[8]

Adoption of a policy of open dialogue therefore threatens to create false and exaggerated expectations. Real dialogue, on the contrary, presupposes the sharing of certain presuppositions and will therefore operate within certain boundaries. The purpose here should be not so much the strengthening of divergent identities, but the development of that kind of identity that can thrive within a Christian healthcare institution. Since the Christian ethical values strongly endorse human dignity, it should be noted that also many non-believers can very much feel at home in a Christian institution where they will find themselves supported in their own vision or vocation.

The objective behind the combination of 'authentic' and 'internal' pluralism is of course a laudable objective: one does not want to approach the current situation with defeatism, but, on the contrary, regard the difficulties of our post-modern situation as opportunities and challenges with the intention to make the best of it. However, especially in a demanding professional environment, it is essential to not losing sight of the original inspiration in order to safeguard the added value of a care that is rooted in a particular spirituality or philosophy of life. Only in this way can interested persons come into contact (again) with a lively Christian tradition that shapes the provision of healthcare in Catholic healthcare institutions. All this is why one can hardly plead for authentic pluralism and at the same time defend the idea of internal pluralism.

---

[8] See G.K. CHESTERTON, *Orthodoxy*, New York, Doubleday (Image Books), 1959, p. 83: "It is extremely difficult for a person to defend something he or she is utterly convinced about". This is because that what really matters is so strongly entangled within a whole network of convictions, attitudes, meanings, and with a whole way of (concrete) living that it seems an endless task to capture that significance in a separate argument, or even to concisely explain the meaning of it. See also H. DE DIJN, *Taboes, monsters en loterijen. Ethiek in de laat-moderne tijd* [Taboos, monsters and lotteries. Ethics in the late modern era], p. 65.

2. Euthanasia within the context of real pluralism

The Belgian lawmaker decided that euthanasia should no longer be penalised when certain conditions are met. Of course, this politico-juridical fact does not by itself mean that euthanasia has become ethically acceptable, nor that this law should be exempt from democratic discussion and criticism, nor that an individual ('subjective') right to euthanasia would exist. Yet the adoption of the law leads many to assume one or more of these views. This shows that laws of this kind are not neutral, pragmatic rules, but expressions of a mentality which in its turn affects people's minds often in unforeseen ways. Within the framework of the current, highly technical and professionally organised healthcare settings, and in combination with all sorts of political and financial pressure, the law swiftly seems to make practising euthanasia — no matter how limited in numbers — perfectly acceptable or self-evident. Therefore one can expect a further broadening of the euthanasia practice to other categories such as minors and people living with dementia. In this regard, the propaganda battle in much of the Belgian media is already raging. It is this situation with the looming danger of 'euthanasiasm'[9] which I want to discuss briefly now.

During the process of approval and implementation of the law on euthanasia an appeal was made to a number of principles and opinions which any right-minded person was supposed to accept. The impression was — and still is — conveyed that a statutory regulation for euthanasia serves a modest and highly dignified purpose: helping terminal patients to end their hopeless suffering and die a merciful death at their own explicit request. At the same time reference was (and is) made to the necessity of respecting the right to self-determination. Finally, the medical act itself was presented as free of any tragedy: it only seems to be a matter of 'giving an injection' or 'pulling the plug' after which the patient will 'go to sleep forever'. Against the background of these assumptions, the opponents of the law were (and are) inevitably portrayed as individuals who, from set

---

[9] I borrow this term from Willem Jan Otten who describes with it a sphere or attitude "in which the tragic, which is always embedded in life, is more and more denied or obliterated"; see W.J. OTTEN, 'De voorstelling van de dood als oplossing' in H. ACHTERHUIS et al. (eds.), Als de dood voor het leven. Over professionele hulp bij zelfmoord [Scared to death by life. On assisted suicide], Amsterdam, Van Oorschot, 1995, p. 61.

religious prejudices, interfere with issues that are none of their business. They also seem to overdramatise the situation by projecting the practice of euthanasia by physicians as the crossing of a fundamental ethical boundary.

Anyone who is capable of only slightly distancing him or herself from a purely partisan position will immediately recognise that we have to do here not with disagreement between liberal-thinking advocates of human dignity and humanity, on the one hand, and obscurantist, ideologically determined heartlessness, on the other. However, it apparently is not very easy to represent the position of opponents of the euthanasia law as they themselves see it, *i.e.* as involving a strong and spontaneous reluctance vis-à-vis the desire of complete control over one's own death (and life). This difficulty is certainly related to the fact that the advocates of euthanasia only need to appeal to a concrete image: the emaciated, bedridden ill person, the terminal patient begging for a merciful death. Opponents on the contrary always seem to need to appeal to abstract ideas such as the sanctity of life or the irreversible nature of life termination. However, it could well be that precisely the kind of principles that the supporters need to appeal to, are the real abstract principles. Which 'self' is the subject of discussion when one speaks of the right to self-determination? What exactly does freedom mean in the terminal phase of people's lives and can one in such instances speak of true self-determination? It may well be the case that precisely those images that spontaneously plead in favour of the law are only convincing because they are isolated and projected on their own, like television images, because human imagination itself is not or no longer able to draw in other images in order to obtain a better or more complete picture. Maybe our powers of imagination and sound judgment fail us while we are carried away by isolated and edited pictures?

The enormous emphasis that is put on self-determination these days and the rejection of any interference by others, whether or not via the law, gives the impression that society has not a single ethical directive to offer its citizens and that those who want to see certain ethical principles represented in the law are not of this day and age. It is however important to realise that the law always inevitably supports specific ethical norms and values: *e.g.* with regard to incest, sadomasochism, cannibalism, man-woman or child-adult relationships, the treatment of dead human bodies, etc. With its near exclusive emphasis on self-determination and quality of life the law on euthanasia also embodies a well-defined message which is anything but neutral, and hard to reconcile with an idea of human dignity that is not reduced to the catering for individual sensitivities.[10] This underlying message is in effect hard to reconcile with the idea that each human life must be respected regardless of its qualities, that human life is not the property of a sole individual or a 'particule élémentaire', as the French writer Michel Houellebecq[11] describes post-modern individuals, but on the contrary an intrinsic part of a network of relations.

The use of so-called obvious principles and innocent pictures is a time-honoured strategy. One so easily speaks of the right to have a child of one's own. Embryo research is projected as perfectly common research into a cluster of cells which, in its early stages, cannot even be regarded as the beginning of an individual entity. However, from a scientific point of view medical research always concerns 'just' a cluster of cells. When dealing with human cells, a cultivated and civilised human sensibility tells us that what scientifically speaking are only gradual differences, may concern essential distinctions when viewed from an ethical standpoint. That is why humans, children, neonates and even embryos deserve special respect; that is why human remains must be treated differently than those of animals. The excessive instrumentalisation and commodification of living or dead human organisms and of reproduction is precisely what racist, fascist and eugenic organisations did to certain groups of people in the course of recent history. Are we now inadvertently on the way to collectively do this to ourselves in the most prosperous countries in the world?

"Having children is not a right, it's a blessing", the saying goes. We have just as little right to die as we have to live or to have children ourselves: each time it involves a gift which we, in awe of the mystery of life, must accept, and sometimes we very much need others since acceptance is not always an easy affair whether in the terminal phase of life or not. Our problem seems to be that nothing seems to inspire awe anymore, neither life nor death. Respect and awe for mystery is not only the business of religious people, it can

[10] I call this reduction 'sentimentalism'; see H. DE DIJN, *De herontdekking van de ziel. Voor een volwaardige kwaliteitszorg* [The rediscovery of the soul. For adequate quality care], Kapellen — Kampen, Pelckmans — Klement, 2002, p. 13 ff.

[11] M. HOUELLEBECQ, *Les particules élémentaires*, Paris, Flammarion, 1998.

also be found among non-believers. Therefore talk about the mystery of life (and death) is not a relic of a superseded Catholicism but a matter of general human sensibility. Greek mythology tells the story of Prometheus who stole the fire of the Gods: the beginning of technology and mastery over nature and life. Zeus, so the story goes, realised how disastrous that possession could be to humankind. Instead of demanding it back, he compensated it with a gift of his own, a two-tiered gift in fact: justice and awe.[12] Without justice and particularly without awe for the mystery of life, without the realisation that mankind is not 'the measure of all things' as Protagoras claimed, technology and science are not a gift, but doom. Mythology here seems to be wiser than philosophy.

Let us once again return to the relationship between imaginative power and euthanasia. One will only realise what really is at stake in the legal regulation of euthanasia when one does not close one's imagination and thought to all sorts of matters which opponents of the law stress, such as the kind of message being sent by the legislature, with its highly symbolic authority, to individuals about the quality and dignity of their lives. What will the disabled, the elderly and their caregivers think of such a message? Human dignity is narrowed down to the ability to have certain experiences and when someone lacks these qualities or experiences their dignity is said to be affected. Respect for human dignity however, is only possible through our imaginative power and judgment that recognises in every human body, no matter how bruised or broken, shrivelled or mutilated it is, a human person and not just an experience machine that can better be written off.[13] Viewed in this way, human dignity is never uniquely determined by the 'quality of life'. Furthermore, should we not urgently start to listen more to caregivers who in their daily professional practice care for people with dementia, to the disabled themselves, on how they regard the law and certain new proposals. After all, they are the real experts. Besides, when we are no longer able to consider the lives of those people as dignified, we will increasingly classify their lives as 'superfluous' and more and more people will consider *themselves* as superfluous. Do we not

[12] See P. WOODRUFF, *Reverence: Renewing a Forgotten Virtue*, Oxford, Oxford University Press, 2001, p. 57.

[13] See H. DE DIJN, *Taboes, monsters en loterijen* [Taboos, monsters and lotteries], chapter 2, pp. 31-52.

realize how easily people, especially young and old people, are led to think that their kinds of lives are no longer worth living: should we give in to their despair? There are so many matters in life which, according to someone's feelings, can be degrading to themselves or others. Will all that become sufficient reason to obtain 'a merciful death'?

Prior to the approval of the Belgian law on euthanasia, the supporters emphatically emphasised that the danger of a slippery slope was a fantasy, fabricated for the sake of opposition to the law. Hardly had the law come into force before some already argued for an extension, so that the law would not only cover life termination for terminal patients, but also for incurable, non-terminal patients, people with dementia or suffering from depression and certain categories of ill or handicapped children. Where all of a sudden is the condition of self-determination? The proponents, who now argue for an extension of the current regulation of termination of life, suggest that any malpractice will be ruled out. However, it is hard to imagine how one can reconcile this claim with the situation of the long-term seriously ill, of depressed and demented people who undoubtedly will experience pressure from family members and financial considerations. And how do healthcare workers have to interpret the meaning of their care for these categories of people once euthanasia is 'self-evident' anyway? Unbearable mental suffering has already been accepted as a sufficient criterion for euthanasia (in Belgium). In this way, the door has been opened for legally permitted assisted suicide. Will the medical corps of the Low Countries soon assist the death wish of all those who are tired of life or who feel their lives to no longer meet the standards of quality and self-management that are not only projected by the media and various other institutions, but now also by the law itself? How can the relationship between caregiver and patient that is primarily based on trust continue to survive in this context? Respect for human dignity cannot simply be equated with compassion, nor is compassion always a good thing (compassion can also be selective, changeable, or a form of hidden self-pity). The question whether the physician's compassion is indeed a good indicator for professional medical behaviour cannot be evaded.[14]

---

[14] On this issue, see H. ACHTERHUIS *et al.* (eds.), *Als de dood voor het leven. Over professionele hulp bij zelfmoord* [Scared to death by life. On assisted suicide], especially F. Koerselman's contribution.

Conclusion

At the very least, real pluralism means that in a society certain groups can organise healthcare or education on the basis of a specific tradition, on the basis of their own religious and/or ethical views. This does not mean that in the institutions concerned all caregivers, let alone all patients, must be firm believers. It is customary today to plead for internal pluralism within such traditionally affiliated institutions. If internal pluralism means that religious and ethical accents are constantly in jeopardy, then it is not desirable. This does not mean that a tradition is exempt of criticism, but this criticism must start from a thorough familiarity with, and respect for, the tradition. C.S. Lewis expresses it as follows: "Outside the *Tao* there is no ground for criticizing either the *Tao* or anything else." "Those who understand the spirit of the *Tao* and who have been led by that spirit can modify it in directions which that spirit itself demands. Only they can know what those directions are. The outsider knows nothing about the matter."[15] An open mindset is something else than the fear of asking others to cooperate with *your* values in their own way. One should not forget that religiously inspired values are not unworldly or inhuman values. On the contrary, reflection will show that religious values are specific interpretations of views that are also held *mutatis mutandis* by people outside those traditions as well.

For the benefit of preserving a humane society it is of the highest importance that within that society the hesitancy towards euthanasia remains. Also within the existent regulatory framework, this can be done in different ways: by giving not only individual doctors and nurses, but also hospitals the right to refuse to cooperate on moral grounds (for the time being it is unclear whether Belgian hospitals have a regulatory basis to appeal to 'conscientious' grounds to refuse the practice of euthanasia within their walls); by suggesting the procedural incorporation of a palliative filter in the law, such as the Association of Care Institutions and the Palliative Care Federation have proposed.

The existence of such procedures is in itself a good thing since they cannot be ignored out of hand. They offer something to hold on to

---

[15] See C.S. LEWIS, *The Abolition of Man*. Glasgow, Collins/Fount Paperback, 1990, p. 30-31. (With *Tao* Lewis means what others mean with the fundamental ethical norms and values of the natural law).

when hard and painful decisions have to be made. Yet, one needs to be vigilant for a real danger which again relates to a lack of imaginative power in a culture where everything is homogenised in an orderly and measurable system. As long as one follows the prescribed procedures, one seems exempted from thinking for oneself and from any personal responsibility. Acting on the basis of such procedures, the ethically unthinkable can easily be interpreted as just another, logical step, although not taken straight away, yet in line with what is already accepted. The way in which procedures and requirements of good practice are formulated and obeyed, can give compliance the aura of doing what is ethically required. We need to realise however that compliance with regulations and fulfilling one's professional duty is not automatically to be equated with acting *ethically*.

When following rules and procedures we need to continue, both individually and as a healthcare team, to respect the mystery of each human life, no matter how miserable its state is; we need to continue to cultivate the powers of ethical imagination and judgment which pay attention to what is awe-inspiring behind or in the life and especially the death of each person. This will not be possible without healthcare workers themselves keeping in touch with some kind of spiritual source of strength, courage and awe.

References

ACHTERHUIS, H., J. GOUD, F. KOERSELMAN, W.J. OTTEN & T. SCHALKEN, *Als de dood voor het leven. Over professionele hulp bij zelfmoord* [Scared to death by life. On assisted-suicide], Amsterdam, Van Oorschot, 1995.

CHESTERTON, G.K., *Orthodoxy*, New York, Doubleday (Image Books), 1959.

DE DIJN, H., 'Tolerance, Loyalty to Values and Respect for the Law' in *Ethical Perspectives* 1/1(1994), pp. 27-32.

DE DIJN, H., *Hoe overleven wij de vrijheid?* [How can we survive liberty?], Kapellen — Kampen, Pelckmans — Kok Agora, 1997.

DE DIJN, H., 'Voorbij de ontzuiling [Beyond depillarisation]' in *Streven* 69:4 (2002), pp. 301-311.

DE DIJN, H., *De herontdekking van de ziel. Voor een volwaardige kwaliteitszorg* [The rediscovery of the soul. For adequate quality care], Kapellen — Kampen, Pelckmans — Klement, 2002.

DE DIJN, H., 'Cultural Identity, Religion, Moral Pluralism and the Law' in *Bijdragen. International Journal in Philosophy and Theology* 64/3(2003), pp. 286-298.

DE DIJN, H., *Taboes, monsters en loterijen. Ethiek in de laat-moderne tijd* [Taboos, monsters and lotteries. Ethics in the late modern era], Kapellen — Kampen, Pelckmans — Klement, 2003.

HOUELLEBECQ, M., *Les particules élémentaires*, Paris, Flammarion, 1998.

LEWIS, C.S., *The Abolition of Man*. Glasgow, Collins/Fount Paperback, 1990.

SCHWALL, H., 'Erfzonde, erfwonde' in *TGL* (Tijdschrift voor Geestelijk Leven) 59/5(2003), pp. 529-541.

VERBOND DER VERZORGINGSINSTELLINGEN, 'Pluralisme en ethische dialoog in christelijke verzorgingsinstellingen [Assocation of care institutions, Pluralism and ethical dialogue in Christian healthcare institutions]', 24 October 2003.

WOODRUFF, P., *Reverence. Renewing a Forgotten Virtue*, Oxford, Oxford University Press, 2001.

ACKNOWLEDGEMENTS

Some of the materials comprising this book have appeared in earlier versions in previous publications, whose editors have kindly granted permission to reprint.

An earlier version of chapter 1 originally appeared in *Medical Law Review*.

> M. ADAMS & H. NYS, 'Comparative reflections on the Belgian Euthanasia Act 2002' in *Medical Law Review* 11(2003), pp. 353-376. Republished by permission of Oxford University Press.

Earlier versions of chapters 2, 4, 5, 8 and 9 appeared in *Ethical Perspectives*.

> BROECKAERT, B. & R. JANSSENS, 'Palliative care and euthanasia: Belgian and Dutch perspectives' in *Ethical Perspectives* 9(2002), pp. 156-175.
>
> WIDDERSHOVEN, G.A.M. 'Beyond autonomy and beneficence: The moral basis of euthanasia in the Netherlands' in *Ethical Perspectives* 9(2002), pp. 96-102.
>
> SULMASY, D.P., 'Death, dignity and the theory of value' in *Ethical Perspectives* 9(2002), pp. 103-130.
>
> JANS, J., 'Christian churches and euthanasia in the Low Countries: Background, argumentation and commentary' in *Ethical Perspectives* 9(2002), pp. 119-133.
>
> GASTMANS, C., 'Caring for a dignified end of life in a Christian healthcare institution: The view of Caritas Catholica Flanders' in *Ethical Perspectives* 9(2002), pp. 134-145.

Chapter 6 originally appeared in *Bijdragen, International Journal in Philosophy and Theology*.

> MEULENBERGS, T. & P. SCHOTSMANS, 'The sanctity of autonomy? Transcending the opposition between a quality of life and a sanctity of life ethic' in *Bijdragen, International Journal in Philosophy and Theology* 62(2001), pp. 280-303.

PERSONALIA

Maurice Adams studied at the Universities of Maastricht, Leuven and Oxford and obtained his Ph.D. in Law at the Catholic University of Leuven (Belgium). Currently, he is professor of law at the University of Antwerp, where he teaches jurisprudence and comparative law. The last few years he has published widely on the relation between law and ethics, especially focusing on the regulation of euthanasia. He advised Belgian parliament on the Euthanasia Act.

Bert Broeckaert studied Religious Sciences and Theology and received his Ph.D. in Theology from the Catholic University of Leuven. From 1998 until 2001, he was post-doctoral researcher at the Centre for Biomedical Ethics and Law (Leuven) focussing on the foundations of medical decisions concerning the end of life. He also served as a core group member of the European Pallium project on palliative care ethics. Currently, he is director of the Interdisciplinary Centre for Religious Studies (Leuven), advisor of the study group ethics of the Federation Palliative Care Flanders and member of the Belgian Advisory Committee on Bioethics.

Roger Burggraeve studied Philosophy in Rome and Theology in Leuven where he received his Ph.D. in Theology in 1980. Currently, he is professor in moral theology in Leuven. He published several works on the ethics and religious thinking of Emmanuel Levinas. His scholarly interests include the relationship between Christian faith and ethics, relational and sexual ethics and education, ethics and pastoral guidance, and the relationship between the bible and philosophy.

Herman De Dijn studied Philosophy at the Catholic University of Leuven and obtained his Doctoral Degree in Philosophy at the same university; did post-doctoral research in Cambridge University (UK). Currently, he is professor of modern philosophy in Leuven and a member of the Royal Belgian Academy of Sciences and Arts. He is the author of international publications mainly on 17th and 18th century philosophy (Spinoza and Hume) and of several philosophical essays (in Dutch) on problems related to contemporary society and culture.

Marta van Dijk studied Health Sciences at the University of Maastricht (the Netherlands). She currently works as an advisor to the House of Care Foundation in Sittard.

Chris Gastmans received a Doctoral Degree in Theology from the Catholic University of Leuven. He is associate professor of medical ethics in the Faculty of Medicine (Centre for Biomedical Ethics and Law) and ethics advisor to the Flemish Association of Care Institutions (Caritas Catholica Vlaanderen). In 2002, he was elected secretary-general of the European Association of Centres for Medical Ethics (EACME). He is teaching and doing research in the field of health care ethics, especially chronic care, palliative care, care for the elderly, nursing ethics and empirical ethics.

Jan Jans obtained a Doctoral Degree in Theology from the Catholic University of Leuven (Belgium). From 1985 until 1990, he was research assistant at the Centre of Biomedical Ethics and Law. Since 1991 he is associate professor of moral theology at Tilburg Faculty of Theology (the Netherlands). He is also visiting professor at St. Augustine College of South Africa. His main areas of scholarly interest include images of God, personalism and ethical methodology, including feminism, intercultural ethics and the ethics of medical technology and electronic media.

Rien Janssens graduated in Theology at the Catholic University of Nijmegen (the Netherlands). Since 1996 he has been working at the department of Ethics, Philosophy and History of Medicine of the University Medical Center St Radboud Nijmegen where he served as a project manager of the European Pallium project on palliative care ethics (1998-2001). In 2001, he successfully defended his thesis 'Palliative care: Concepts and ethics'. Currently, he is working as a senior researcher at the University of Nijmegen where he studies the empirical and ethical aspects of palliative sedation.

Agnes M. Meershoek studied Health Sciences at the University of Maastricht, where she also obtained her Doctoral Degree. Currently, she is lecturer at the same university and is doing research into normative aspects of Sickness and Disability arrangements.

Tom Meulenbergs read Philosophy at the Institute of Philosophy, Catholic University of Leuven, where he earned his Master of Arts in Philosophy. From 2000 until 2004, he was a researcher at the Centre for Biomedical Ethics and Law (Leuven). Currently, he is working as a policy advisor on health care for the Ministry of Flanders and is researching for a Ph.D. in Social Health Sciences on the subject of health care ethics committees and innovative forms of ethics support in clinical settings.

Herman Nys obtained a Doctoral degree in Law at the Catholic University of Leuven and specialised in medical law at the Universities of Nijmegen and London. He is professor of medical law at the Catholic University of Leuven and professor in international health law at the University of Maastricht. His main research interests are genetics, biomedical research with human beings and end of life issues. He advised Belgian parliament on the Euthanasia Bill.

Paul Schotsmans studied Educational Sciences and obtained a Doctoral Degree in Theology at the Catholic University of Leuven. He is professor of medical ethics at the Catholic University of Leuven and director of the Centre for Biomedical Ethics and Law. He also serves as a member in the Belgian Advisory Committee on Bioethics, a board member of the International Association of Bioethics and is president of the European Association of Centres of Medical Ethics (EACME). He advised Belgian parliament on the Euthanasia Bill.

Daniel P. Sulmasy is a Franciscan Friar who holds the Sisters of Charity Chair in Ethics at St. Vincent's Hospital (Manhattan), and serves as professor of medicine and director of the Bioethics Institute of New York Medical College, Valhalla (New York). He received his A.B. and M.D. degrees from Cornell University and completed his residency, chief residency, and postdoctoral fellowship at the Johns Hopkins Hospital. He received his Ph.D. in Philosophy from Georgetown University in 1995. His books include *The Healer's Calling* and *Methods in Medical Ethics*. He also serves as editor-inchief of the journal *Theoretical Medicine and Bioethics*.

Guy A.M. Widdershoven studied Philosophy, Political Sciences and Mathematics at the University of Amsterdan (the Netherlands) where he obtained his Doctoral Degree in Philosophy. Currently, he is Professor of Health Care Ethics at Maastricht University and president of the European Association of Centres for Medical Ethics (EACME). His main research interests are ethics of chronic care, especially care for the elderly, psychiatric care, empirical ethics, and hermeneutic ethics.

APPENDIX I

THE BELGIAN ACT ON EUTHANASIA
OF 28 MAY 2002*

ALBERT II, King of the Belgians,
To all those present now and in the future, greetings.
The Chambers have approved and We sanction what follows:

Section 1

This law governs a matter provided in article 78 of the Constitution.

Chapter I: General provisions

Section 2

For the purposes of this Act, euthanasia is defined as intentionally terminating life by someone other than the person concerned, at the latter's request.

Chapter II: Conditions and procedure

Section 3

§1. The physician who performs euthanasia commits no criminal offence when he/she ensures that:

- the patient has attained the age of majority or is an emancipated minor, and is legally competent and conscious at the moment of making the request;
- the request is voluntary, well-considered and repeated, and is not the result of any external pressure;

---

* Translation provided by Dale Kidd (European Centre for Ethics, Catholic University of Leuven) under the scientific supervision of Prof. Herman Nys, Centre for Biomedical Ethics and Law, Faculty of Medicine, Catholic University of Leuven (Belgium).

– the patient is in a medically futile condition of constant and unbearable physical or mental suffering that can not be alleviated, resulting from a serious and incurable disorder caused by illness or accident;

and when he/she has respected the conditions and procedures as provided in this Act.

§2. Without prejudice to any additional conditions imposed by the physician on his/her own action, before carrying out euthanasia he/she must in each case:

1) inform the patient about his/her health condition and life expectancy, discuss with the patient his/her request for euthanasia and the possible therapeutic and palliative courses of action and their consequences. Together with the patient, the physician must come to the belief that there is no reasonable alternative to the patient's situation and that the patient's request is completely voluntary;

2) be certain of the patient's constant physical or mental suffering and of the durable nature of his/her request. To this end, the physician has several conversations with the patient spread out over a reasonable period of time, taking into account the progress of the patient's condition;

3) consult another physician about the serious and incurable character of the disorder and inform him/her about the reasons for this consultation. The physician consulted reviews the medical record, examines the patient and must be certain of the patient's constant and unbearable physical or mental suffering that cannot be alleviated. The physician consulted reports on his/her findings.

The physician consulted must be independent of the patient as well as of the attending physician and must be competent to give an opinion about the disorder in question. The attending physician informs the patient about the results of this consultation;

4) if there is a nursing team that has regular contact with the patient; discuss the request of the patient with the nursing team or its members,

5) if the patient so desires, discuss his/her request with relatives appointed by the patient;

6) be certain that the patient has had the opportunity to discuss his/her request with the persons that he/she wanted to meet.

§3. If the physician believes the patient is clearly not expected to die in the near future, he/she must also:

1) consult a second physician, who is a psychiatrist or a specialist in the disorder in question, and inform him/her of the reasons for such a consultation. The physician consulted reviews the medical record, examines the patient and must ensure himself about the constant and unbearable physical or mental suffering that cannot be alleviated, and of the voluntary, well-considered and repeated character of the euthanasia request. The physician consulted reports on his/her findings. The physician consulted must be independent of the patient as well as of the physician initially consulted. The physician informs the patient about the results of this consultation;

2) allow at least one month between the patient's written request and the act of euthanasia.

§4. The patient's request must be in writing. The document is drawn up, dated and signed by the patient himself/herself. If the patient is not capable of doing this, the document is drawn up by a person designated by the patient. This person must have attained the age of majority and must not have any material interest in the death of the patient.

This person indicates that the patient is incapable of formulating his/her request in writing and the reasons why. In such a case the request is drafted in the presence of the physician whose name is mentioned on the document. This document must be annexed to the medical record.

The patient may revoke his/her request at any time, in which case the document is removed from the medical record and returned to the patient.

§5. All the requests formulated by the patient, as well as any actions by the attending physician and their results, including the report(s) of the consulted physician(s), are regularly noted in the patient's medical record.

Chapter III: The advance directive

Section 4

§1. In cases where one is no longer able to express one's will, every legally competent person of age, or emancipated minor, can draw up an advance directive instructing a physician to perform euthanasia if the physician ensures that:

– the patient suffers from a serious and incurable disorder, caused by illness or accident;
– the patient is no longer conscious;
– this condition is irreversible given the current state of medical science.

In the advance directive, one or more person(s) taken in confidence can be designated in order of preference, who inform(s) the attending physician about the patient's will. Each person taken in confidence replaces his or her predecessor as mentioned in the advance directive, in the case of refusal, hindrance, incompetence or death. The patient's attending physician, the physician consulted and the members of the nursing team may not act as persons taken in confidence.

The advance directive may be drafted at any moment. It must be composed in writing in the presence of two witnesses, at least one of whom has no material interest in the death of the patient and it must be dated and signed by the drafter, the witnesses and by the person(s) taken in confidence, if applicable.

If a person who wishes to draft an advance directive is permanently physically incapable of writing and signing an advance directive, he/she may designate a person who is of age, and who has no material interest in the death of the person in question, to draft the request in writing, in the presence of two witnesses who have attained the age of majority and at least one of whom has no material interest in the patient's death. The advance directive indicates that the person in question is incapable of signing and why. The advance directive must be dated and signed by the drafter, by the witnesses and by the person(s) taken in confidence, if applicable.

A medical certificate must be annexed to the advance directive proving that the person in question is permanently physically incapable of drafting and signing the advance directive.

An advance directive is only valid if it is drafted or confirmed no more than five years prior to the person's loss of the ability to express his/her wishes.

The advance directive may be amended or revoked at any time.

The King determines the manner in which the advance directive is drafted, registered and confirmed or revoked, and the manner in which it is communicated to the physicians involved via the offices of the National Register.

§2. The physician who performs euthanasia, in consequence of an advance directive as referred to in §1, commits no criminal offence when he ensures that:

 – the patient suffers from a serious and incurable disorder, caused by illness or accident;
 – the patient is unconscious;
 – and this condition is irreversible given the current state of medical science;

and when he/she has respected the conditions and procedures as provided in this Act.

Without prejudice to any additional conditions imposed by the physician on his/her own action, before carrying out euthanasia he/she must:

1) consult another physician about the irreversibility of the patient's medical condition and inform him/her about the reasons for this consultation. The physician consulted consults the medical record and examines the patient. He/she reports on his/her findings.

   When the advance directive names a person taken in confidence, the latter will be informed about the results of this consultation by the attending physician.

   The physician consulted must be independent of the patient as well as of the attending physician and must be competent to give an opinion about the disorder in question;

2) if there is a nursing team that has regular contact with the patient, discuss the content of the advance directive with that team or its members;

3) if a person taken in confidence is designated in the advance directive, discuss the request with that person;

4) if a person taken in confidence is designated in the advance directive, discuss the content of the advance directive with the relatives of the patient designated by the person taken in confidence.

The advance directive, as well as all actions by the attending physician and their results, including the report of the consulted physician, are regularly noted in the patient's medical record.

Chapter IV: Notification

Section 5

Any physician who has performed euthanasia is required to fill in a registration form, drawn up by the Federal Control and Evaluation Commission established by section 6 of this Act, and to deliver this document to the Commission within four working days.

Chapter V: The Federal Control and Evaluation Commission

Section 6

§1. For the implementation of this Act, a Federal Control and Evaluation Commission is established, hereafter referred to as "the commission".

§2. The commission is composed of sixteen members, appointed on the basis of their knowledge and experience in the issues belonging to the commission's jurisdiction. Eight members are doctors of medicine, of whom at least four are professors at a university in Belgium. Four members are professors of law at a university in Belgium, or practising lawyers. Four members are drawn from groups that deal with the problem of incurably ill patients. Membership in the commission cannot be combined with a post in one of the legislative bodies or with a post as a member of the federal government or one of the regional or community governments.

While respecting language parity — where each linguistic group has at least three candidates of each sex — and ensuring pluralistic representation, the members of the commission are appointed by royal decree enacted after deliberation in the Council of Ministers for a four-year term, which may be extended, from a double list of candidates put forward by the Senate. A member's mandate is terminated *de jure* if the member loses the capacity on the basis of which he/she is appointed. The candidates not appointed as sitting members are appointed as substitutes, in the order determined by a list. The commission is chaired by a Dutch-speaking and a French-speaking member. These chairpersons are elected by the commission members of the respective linguistic group.

The commission's decisions are only valid if there is a quorum present of two-thirds of the members.

§3. The commission establishes its own internal regulations.

Section 7

The commission drafts a registration form that must be filled in by the physician whenever he/she performs euthanasia. This document consists of two parts. The first part must be placed under seal by the physician. It includes the following information:

1) the patient's full name and address;
2) the full name, address and health insurance institute registration number of the attending physician;
3) the full name, address and health insurance institute registration number of the physician(s) consulted about the euthanasia request;
4) the full name, address and capacity of all persons consulted by the attending physician, and the date of these consultations;
5) if there exists an advance directive in which one or more persons taken in confidence are designated, the full name of such person(s).

The document's first part is confidential, and is supplied to the commission by the physician. It can only be consulted following a decision by the commission. Under no circumstances the commission may use this document for its evaluation.

The second part is also confidential. It includes the following information:

1) the patient's sex, date of birth and place of birth;
2) the date, time and place of death;
3) the nature of the serious and incurable condition, caused by accident or illness, from which the patient suffered;
4) the nature of the constant and unbearable suffering;
5) the reasons why this suffering could not be alleviated;
6) the elements underlying the assurance that the request is voluntary, well-considered and repeated, and not the result of any external pressure;
7) whether one can expect that the patient would die within the foreseeable future;
8) whether an advance directive has been drafted;
9) the procedure followed by the physician;
10) the capacity of the physician(s) consulted, the recommendations and the information from these consultations;
11) the capacity of the persons consulted by the physician, and the date of these consultations;
12) the manner in which euthanasia was performed and the pharmaceuticals used.

Section 8

The commission studies the completed registration form submitted to it by the attending physician. On the basis of the second part of the registration form, the commission determines whether the euthanasia was performed in accordance with the conditions and the procedure stipulated in this Act. In cases of doubt, the commission may decide by simple majority to revoke anonymity and examine the first part of the registration form. The commission may request the attending physician to provide any information from the medical record having to do with the euthanasia.

The commission hands down a verdict within two months.

If, in a decision taken with a two-thirds majority, the commission is of the opinion that the conditions laid down in this Act have not been fulfilled, then it turns the case over to the public prosecutor of the jurisdiction in which the patient died.

If, after anonymity has been revoked, facts or circumstances come to light which would compromise the independence or impartiality of one of the commission members, this member will have an opportunity to explain or to be challenged during the discussion of this matter in the commission.

Section 9

For the benefit of the legislative chambers, the commission will draft the following reports, the first time within two years of this Act's coming into force and every two years thereafter:

a) a statistical report processing the information from the second part of the completed registration forms submitted by physicians pursuant to section 8;

b) a report in which the implementation of the law is indicated and evaluated;

c) if required, recommendations that could lead to new legislation or other measures concerning the execution of this Act.

For the purpose of carrying out this task, the commission may seek additional information from the various public services and institutions. The information thus gathered is confidential. None of these documents may reveal the identities of any persons named in the dossiers submitted to the commission for the purposes of the review as determined in section 8.

The commission can decide to supply statistical and purely technical data, purged of any personal information, to university research teams that submit a reasoned request for such data.

The commission can grant hearings to experts.

Section 10

The King places an administration at the commission's disposal in order to carry out its legal functions. The composition and language framework of the administrative personnel are established by royal decree, following consultation in the Council of Ministers, on the recommendation of the Minister of Health and the Minister of Justice.

Section 11

The commission's operating costs and personnel costs, including remuneration for its members, are divided equally between the budget of the Minister of Health and the budget of the Minister of Justice.

Section 12

Any person who is involved, in whatever capacity, in implementing this Act is required to maintain confidentiality regarding the information provided to him/her in the exercise of his/her function. He/she is subject to section 458 of the Penal Code.

Section 13

Within six months of submitting the first report and the commission's recommendations referred to in section 9, if any, a debate is to be held in the Chambers of Parliament. The six-month period is suspended during the time that Parliament is dissolved and/or during the time there is no government having the confidence of Parliament.

Chapter VI: Special Provisions

Section 14

The request and the advance directive referred to in sections 3 and 4 of this Act are not compulsory in nature.

No physician may be compelled to perform euthanasia.

No other person may be compelled to assist in performing euthanasia.

Should the physician consulted refuse to perform euthanasia, then he/she must inform the patient and the persons taken in confidence, if any, of this fact in a timely manner, and explain his/her reasons for such refusal. If the refusal is based on medical reasons, then these reasons are noted in the patient's medical record.

At the request of the patient or the person taken in confidence, the physician who refuses to perform euthanasia must communicate the patient's medical record to the physician designated by the patient or person taken in confidence.

Section 15

Any person who dies as a result of euthanasia performed in accordance with the conditions established by this Act is deemed to have died of natural causes for the purposes of contracts he/she had entered into, in particular insurance contracts.

The provisions of section 909 of the Civil Code apply to the members of the nursing team referred to in section 3 of this Act.

Section 16

This Act comes into force no later than three months following publication in the *Official Belgian Gazette*.

Promulgate the present Act, order that it be sealed with the seal of the State and published in the *Official Belgian Gazette*.

Issued at Brussels, 28th May 2002.

ALBERT

for the King:
the Minister of Justice,
M. VERWILGHEN
sealed with the seal of the State:
the Minister of Justice,
M. VERWILGHEN

APPENDIX II

THE DUTCH TERMINATION OF LIFE ON REQUEST AND ASSISTED SUICIDE (REVIEW PROCEDURES) ACT*

Amended legislative proposal

28 November 2000

We BEATRIX, by the grace of God, Queen of the Netherlands, Princess of Orange-Nassau, etc., etc. etc.

Greetings to all who shall see or hear these presents! Be it known:
Whereas We have considered that it is desired to include a ground for exemption from criminal liability for the physician who with due observance of the requirements of due care to be laid down by law terminates a life on request or assists in a suicide of another person, and to provide a statutory notification and review procedure;

We, therefore, having heard the Council of State, and in consultation with the States General, have approved and decreed as We hereby approve and decree:

Chapter I. Definitions of Terms

Article 1

For the purposes of this Act:

a. Our Ministers mean the Ministers of Justice and of Health, Welfare and Sports;
b. assisted suicide means intentionally assisting in a suicide of another person or procuring for that other person the means referred to in Article 294 second paragraph second sentence of the Penal Code;
c. the physician means the physician who according to the notification has terminated a life on request or assisted in a suicide;

---

* Official translation provided by the Dutch Departments of Justice and Foreign Affairs, to be found at *http://www.justitie.nl* and *http://www.minbuza.nl*.

d. the consultant means the physician who has been consulted with respect to the intention by the physician to terminate a life on request or to assist in a suicide;

e. the providers of care mean the providers of care referred to in Article 446 first paragraph of Book 7 of the Civil Code (*Burgerlijk Wetboek*);

f. the committee means a regional review committee referred to in Article 3;

g. the regional inspector means the regional inspector of the Health Care Inspectorate of the Public Health Supervisory Service.

Chapter II. Requirements of Due Care

Article 2

1. The requirements of due care, referred to in Article 293 second paragraph Penal Code mean that the physician:

   a. holds the conviction that the request by the patient was voluntary and well-considered,

   b. holds the conviction that the patient's suffering was lasting and unbearable,

   c. has informed the patient about the situation he was in and about his prospects,

   d. and the patient hold the conviction that there was no other reasonable solution for the situation he was in,

   e. has consulted at least one other, independent physician who has seen the patient and has given his written opinion on the requirements of due care, referred to in parts a — d, and

   f. has terminated a life or assisted in a suicide with due care.

2. If the patient aged sixteen years or older is no longer capable of expressing his will, but prior to reaching this condition was deemed to have a reasonable understanding of his interests and has made a written statement containing a request for termination of life, the physician may carry out this request. The requirements of due care, referred to in the first paragraph, apply *mutatis mutandis*.

3. If the minor patient has attained an age between sixteen and eighteen years and may be deemed to have a reasonable understanding of his interests, the physician may carry out the patient's request for termination of life or assisted suicide, after the parent or the parents exercising parental authority and/or his guardian have been involved in the decision process.

4. If the minor patient is aged between twelve and sixteen years and may be deemed to have a reasonable understanding of his interests, the physician may carry out the patient's request, provided always that the parent

or the parents exercising parental authority and/or his guardian agree with the termination of life or the assisted suicide. The second paragraph applies *mutatis mutandis*.

Chapter III. The Regional Review Committees for Termination of Life on Request and Assisted Suicide

Paragraph 1: Establishment, composition and appointment

Article 3

1. There are regional committees for the review of notifications of cases of termination of life on request and assistance in a suicide as referred to in Article 293 second paragraph or 294 second paragraph second sentence, respectively, of the Penal Code.

2. A committee is composed of an uneven number of members, including at any rate one legal specialist, also chairman, one physician and one expert on ethical or philosophical issues

3. The committee also contains deputy members of each of the categories listed in the first sentence.

Article 4

1. The chairman and the members, as well as the deputy members are appointed by Our Ministers for a period of six years. They may be re-appointed one time for another period of six years.

2. A committee has a secretary and one or more deputy secretaries, all legal specialists, appointed by Our Ministers. The secretary has an advisory role in the committee meetings.

3. The secretary may solely be held accountable by the committee for his activities for the committee.

Paragraph 2: Dismissal

Article 5

Our Ministers may at any time dismiss the chairman and the members, as well as the deputy members at their own request.

Article 6

Our Ministers may dismiss the chairman and the members, as well as the deputy members for reasons of unsuitability or incompetence or for other important reasons.

Paragraph 3: Remuneration

Article 7

The chairman and the members, as well as the deputy members receive a holiday allowance as well as a reimbursement of the travel and accommodation expenses according to the existing government scheme insofar as these expenses are not otherwise reimbursed from the State Funds.

Paragraph 4: Duties and powers

Article 8

1. The committee assesses on the basis of the report referred to in Article 7 second paragraph of the Burial and Cremation Act whether the hysician who has terminated a life on request or assisted in a suicide has acted in accordance with the requirements of due care, referred to in Article 2.

2. The committee may request the physician to supplement his report in writing or verbally, where this is necessary for a proper assessment of the physician's actions.

3. The committee may make enquiries at the municipal autopsist, the consultant or the providers of care involved where this is necessary for a proper assessment of the physician's actions.

Article 9

1. The committee informs the physician within six weeks of the receipt of the report referred to in Article 8 first paragraph in writing of its motivated opinion.

2. The committee informs the Board of Procurators General and the regional health care inspector of its opinion:

   a. if the committee is of the opinion that the physician has failed to act in accordance with the requirements of due care, referred to in Article 2; or
   b. if a situation occurs as referred to in Article 12, final sentence of the Burial and Cremation Act.

   The committee shall inform the physician of this.

3. The term referred to in the first paragraph may be extended one time by a maximum period of six weeks. The committee shall inform the physician of this.

4. The committee may provide a further, verbal explanation on its opinion to the physician. This verbal explanation may take place at the request of the committee or at the request of the physician.

Article 10

The committee is obliged to provide all information to the public prosecutor, at his request, which he may need:

1º for the benefit of the assessment of the physician's actions in the case referred to in Article 9 second paragraph; or

2º for the benefit of a criminal investigation.

The committee shall inform the physician of any provision of information to the public prosecutor.

Paragraph 6: Working method

Article 11

The committee shall ensure the registration of the cases of termination of life or assisted suicide reported for assessment. Further rules on this may be laid down by a ministerial regulation by Our Ministers.

Article 12

1. An opinion is adopted by a simple majority of votes.

2. An opinion may only be adopted by the committee provided all committee members have participated in the vote.

Article 13

At least twice a year, the chairmen of the regional review committees conduct consultations with one another with respect to the working method and the performance of the committees. A representative of the Board of Procurators General and a representative of the Health Care Inspectorate of the Public Health Supervisory Service are invited to attend these consultations.

Paragraph 7: Secrecy and exemption

Article 14

The members and deputy members of the committee are under an obligation of secrecy to keep confidential any information acquired in the performance of their duties, except where any statutory regulation obliges them to divulge this information or where the necessity to divulge information ensues from their duties.

Article 15

A member of the committee that serves on the committee in the treatment of a case exempts himself and may be challenged if there are facts or circumstances that may affect the impartiality of his opinion.

Article 16

A member, a deputy member and the secretary of the committee refrain from rendering an opinion on the intention by a physician to terminate a life on request or to assist in a suicide.

Paragraph 8: Report

Article 17

1. Not later than 1 April, the committees issue a joint annual report to Our Ministers on the activities of the past calendar year. Our Ministers shall lay down a model for this by means of a ministerial regulation.

2. The report on the activities referred to in the first paragraph shall at any rate include the following:

   a. the number of reported cases of termination of life on request and assisted suicide on which the committee has rendered an opinion;
   b. the nature of these cases;
   c. the opinions and the considerations involved.

Article 18

Annually, at the occasion of the submission of the budget to the States General, Our Ministers shall issue a report with respect to the performance of the committees further to the report on the activities as referred to in Article 17 first paragraph.

Article 19

1. On the recommendation of Our Ministers, rules shall be laid down by order in council regarding the committees with respect to

   a. their number and their territorial jurisdiction;
   b. their domicile.

2. Our Ministers may lay down further rules by or pursuant to an order in council regarding the committees with respect to

   a. their size and composition;
   b. their working method and reports.

Chapter IV. Amendments to other Acts

Article 20

The Penal Code shall be amended as follows:

A.

Article 293 shall read:

Article 293

1. A person who terminates the life of another person at that other person's express and earnest request is liable to a term of imprisonment of not more than twelve years or a fine of the fifth category.

2. The offence referred to in the first paragraph shall not be punishable if it has been committed by a physician who has met the requirements of due care as referred to in Article 2 of the Termination of Life on Request and Assisted Suicide (Review Procedures) Act and who informs the municipal autopsist of this in accordance with Article 7 second paragraph of the Burial and Cremation Act.

B.

Article 294 shall read:

Article 294

1. A person who intentionally incites another to commit suicide, is liable to a term of imprisonment of not more than three years or a fine of the fourth category, where the suicide ensues.

2. A person who intentionally assists in the suicide of another or procures for that other person the means to commit suicide, is liable to a term of imprisonment of not more than three years or a fine of the fourth category, where the suicide ensues. Article 293 second paragraph applies *mutatis mutandis*.

C. In Article 295, the following is inserted after '293': first paragraph.

D. In Article 422, the following is inserted after '293': first paragraph.

Article 21

The Burial and Cremation Act shall be amended as follows:

A.

Article 7 shall read:

Article 7

1. A person who has performed a postmortem shall issue a death certificate if he is convinced that death has occurred as a result of a natural cause.

2. If the death was the result of the application of termination of life on request or assisted suicide as referred to in Article 293 second paragraph or Article 294 second paragraph second sentence, respectively, of the Penal Code, the attending physician shall not issue a death certificate and shall promptly notify the municipal autopsist or one of the municipal autopsists of the cause of death by completing a form. The physician shall supplement this form with a reasoned report with respect to the due observance of the requirements of due care referred to in Article 2 of the Termination of Life on Request and Assisted Suicide (Review Procedures) act.

3. If the attending physician in other cases than referred to in the second paragraph believes that he may not issue a death certificate, he must promptly notify the municipal autopsist or one of the municipal autopsists of this by completing a form.

B.

Article 9 shall read:

Article 9

1. The form and the set-up of the models of the death certificate to be issued by the attending physician and by the municipal autopsist shall be laid down by order in council.

2. The form and the set-up of the models of the notification and the report referred to in Article 7 second paragraph, of the notification referred to in Article 7 third paragraph and of the forms referred to in Article 10 first and second paragraph shall be laid down by order in council on the recommendation of Our Minister of Justice and Our Minister of Health, Welfare and Sports.

C.

Article 10 shall read:

Article 10

1. If the municipal autopsist is of the opinion that he cannot issue a death certificate, he shall promptly report this to the public prosecutor by completing a form and he shall promptly notify the registrar of births, deaths and marriages.

2. In the event of a notification as referred to in Article 7 second paragraph and without prejudice to the first paragraph, the municipal autopsist shall promptly report to the regional review committee referred to in Article 3 of the Termination of Life on Request and Assisted Suicide (Review Procedures) Act by completing a form. He shall enclose a reasoned report as referred to in Article 7 second paragraph.

D.

The following sentence shall be added to Article 12, reading: If the public prosecutor, in the cases referred to in Article 7 second paragraph, is of the opinion that he cannot issue a certificate of no objection against the burial or cremation, he shall promptly inform the municipal autopsist and the regional review committee referred to in Article 3 of the Termination of Life on Request and Assisted Suicide (Review Procedures) Act of this.

E.

In Article 81, first part, '7, first paragraph' shall be replaced by '7, first and second paragraph'.

Article 22

The General Administrative Law Act (*Algemene wet bestuursrecht*) shall be amended as follows: At the end of part d of Article 1:6, the full stop shall be replaced by a semicolon and the following shall be added to the fifth part, reading:

    e. decisions and actions in the implementation of the Termination of Life and Assisted Suicide (Review Procedures) Act.

Chapter V. Final Provisions

Article 23

This Act shall take effect as of a date to be determined by Royal Decree.

Article 24

This Act may be cited as: Termination of Life on Request and Assisted Suicide (Review Procedures) Act.

We hereby order and command that this Act shall be published in the *Bulletin of Acts and Decrees* and that all ministerial departments, authorities, bodies and officials whom it may concern shall diligently implement it.

Done

The Minister of Justice,

The Minister of Health, Welfare and Sports.
Upper House, parliamentary year 2000-2001, 26 691, no 137

PRINTED ON PERMANENT PAPER • IMPRIME SUR PAPIER PERMANENT • GEDRUKT OP DUURZAAM PAPIER - ISO 9706

N.V. PEETERS S.A., WAROTSTRAAT 50, B-3020 HERENT